THE ULTIMATE AUTOIMMUNE PROTOCOL DIET COOKBOOK

120+ Easy and Satisfying Recipes to Reclaim Your Health

DR. GILMAR

CONTENTS.

Welcome to The Ultimate Autoimmune Protocol Diet Cookbook.

This book is a beginners' guide to the autoimmune protocol diet (AIP). If you have this book in your hands, you may be on a path of regaining your well-being and vigor. Maybe you are going through autoimmune disease, or you want relief from chronic inflammation, or even you just want your overall health improved. Whichever it is, this is the best place for you.

What's the Autoimmune Protocol (AIP) Diet?

The autoimmune protocol (AIP) diet helps in identifying and eliminating any foods that could potentially cause inflammation and autoimmune responses in your body. It is founded on an understanding that some types of food can contribute to leaky gut syndrome, dysbiosis and immune system dysregulation which are all common causes of autoimmune diseases.

Why Choose AIP Diet?

Unlike other diets which are focused only on weight loss or general health improvement; AIP diet addresses specific needs of individuals with autoimmunity. This diet aims at minimizing symptoms by avoiding potentially inflammatory foods while embracing healing nutrient-dense ones for increased quality of life and faster recovery.

What is the Mechanism of Action for the AIP Diet?

For example, it removes some foods that are widely known to be problematic for many people like grains, dairy products, legumes, processed food and refined sugar which brings inflammation. This makes it possible to heal your body thus reducing the levels of swelling that can cause autoimmune symptoms at times.

What Will You Get from this Cookbook?

The following recipes have been compiled in this book while taking keen note on AIP diet recommendations. They range from comforting soups and stews to hearty main courses and tasty desserts meant to nourish you and promote your recovery process.

How to Use This Cookbook.

Whether you're a beginner in AIP or an old hand with it, this cookbook has something in store for everybody. Further, each recipe includes information about any adjustments or substitutes necessary so as to fit individual tastes. Besides, we include a practical meal planning guide along with a grocery list that will assist you in staying organized when shopping.

Final Thoughts.

The Autoimmune Protocol Diet Cookbook (AIP) is not just a recipe book; it's a guide to better health and happiness. We're with you every step of the way on your AIP journey and glad to be part of your healing process. So, put on your apron, grab your knives and let's get cooking!

INTRODUCTION.

What is AIP Diet?

The AIP Diet is a specialized version of the Paleo diet, designed to help people with autoimmune conditions reduce inflammation, heal their gut, and manage symptoms. It's not just about what you eat; it's a holistic approach that considers lifestyle factors, stress management, and sleep quality.

When you have an autoimmune disease, your immune system mistakenly attacks healthy cells in your body, leading to chronic inflammation and various symptoms. The AIP Diet aims to identify and eliminate foods that might trigger this immune response, while also focusing on nutrient-dense foods that support healing and gut health.

How does AIP Diet work?

The AIP Diet works by removing foods that are known to cause inflammation and gut irritation, while also emphasizing nutrient-rich foods that support your body's healing processes. Here's how it works in a nutshell:

1. **Elimination Phase:** During the initial phase of the AIP Diet, you'll eliminate potentially inflammatory foods such as grains, dairy, eggs, legumes, nuts, seeds, nightshade vegetables, processed foods, and refined sugars. This phase typically lasts for a minimum of 30 days, but some people may need to extend it based on their symptoms and health goals.

2. **Reintroduction Phase:** After the elimination phase, you'll gradually reintroduce eliminated foods one at a time, monitoring your body's response to each food. This phase helps you identify which foods trigger your symptoms and which ones are safe for you to eat.

3. **Personalization:** Once you've identified your trigger foods, you can personalize your AIP Diet to suit your body's needs. This might involve continuing to avoid certain foods, while others may be able to reintroduce more foods back into their diet.

4. **Lifestyle Factors:** In addition to diet, the AIP protocol emphasizes the importance of lifestyle factors such as stress management, adequate sleep, and regular physical activity. These factors play a crucial role in supporting your immune system and overall health.

5. **Nutrient-Dense Foods:** The AIP Diet focuses on nutrient-dense foods such as vegetables, fruits, grass-fed meats, wild-caught fish, healthy fats, and fermented foods. These foods provide essential vitamins, minerals, antioxidants, and anti-inflammatory compounds that support healing and gut health.

By following the AIP Diet, you're not only changing what you eat but also how you live. It's a journey of self-discovery and empowerment, where you take control of your health and well-being. Remember, it's not just about the destination; it's about the journey and the positive changes you make along the way.

Benefits of the AIP Diet.

The AIP Diet offers a wide range of benefits for those with autoimmune conditions and beyond. Here are some of the key benefits you can expect:

1. **Reduced Inflammation:** By eliminating inflammatory foods and focusing on nutrient-dense foods, the AIP Diet can help reduce inflammation in the body, which is crucial for managing autoimmune conditions.

2. **Improved Gut Health:** The AIP Diet emphasizes gut-healing foods such as bone broth, fermented vegetables, and collagen-rich foods, which can support the health of your gut lining and improve digestion.

3. **Better Nutrient Absorption:** By removing foods that can cause gut irritation and inflammation, the AIP Diet can help improve nutrient absorption, ensuring your body gets the vitamins and minerals it needs for optimal health.

4. **Balanced Blood Sugar Levels:** The AIP Diet encourages the consumption of whole, unprocessed foods, which can help stabilize blood sugar levels and reduce cravings for sugary foods.

5. **Weight Management:** Many people find that the AIP Diet helps them maintain a healthy weight, as it focuses on whole, nutrient-dense foods and eliminates processed foods that can contribute to weight gain.

6. **Improved Energy Levels:** By providing your body with the nutrients it needs and reducing inflammation, the AIP Diet can help improve your energy levels and overall vitality.

7. **Better Mood and Mental Clarity:** Some people report improvements in mood and mental clarity when following the

AIP Diet, which may be due to the removal of foods that can negatively affect brain function.

Foods to Include and Exclude in AIP Diet.

The AIP Diet focuses on whole, nutrient-dense foods while eliminating potentially inflammatory foods. Here's a general guideline of foods to include and exclude:

Foods to Include:

- Vegetables (except nightshades)

- Fruits

- Quality meats (grass-fed, pasture-raised)

- Fish and seafood (wild-caught)

- Healthy fats (coconut oil, olive oil, avocado)

- Bone broth

- Fermented foods (sauerkraut, kimchi)

- Herbs and spices

Foods to Exclude:

- Grains (wheat, barley, oats, rice, etc.)

- Dairy products

- Legumes (beans, lentils, peanuts)

- Nightshade vegetables (tomatoes, peppers, eggplant, potatoes)

- Eggs

- Nuts and seeds

- Processed foods

- Refined sugars and sweeteners

- Seed oils (canola, soybean, sun flower)

Remember, the AIP Diet is not a one-size-fits-all approach. It's important to listen to your body and make adjustments based on your individual needs and health goals. The goal is to support your body's natural healing process and improve your overall health and well-being.

Tips for Starting and Sticking to the AIP Diet.

Starting a new diet can be challenging, but with the right mindset and strategies, you can set yourself up for success on the AIP diet

Here are some tips to help you get started and stay committed:

1. **Educate Yourself:** Take the time to understand the principles behind the AIP diet and why certain foods are eliminated and others are encouraged. This will help you make informed choices and stay motivated.

2. **Plan Ahead:** Planning is key to success on the AIP diet. Spend some time each week meal planning, grocery

shopping, and preparing meals in advance. This will help you avoid last-minute temptations and stay on track.

3. **Start Slowly:** Transitioning to the AIP diet can be overwhelming, especially if you're used to eating a different way. Start by gradually eliminating one food group at a time and replacing them with AIP-friendly alternatives.

4. **Get Creative in the Kitchen:** The AIP diet doesn't have to be boring! Experiment with different herbs, spices, and cooking methods to keep your meals interesting and flavorful.

5. **Find Support:** Joining a community of others who are following the AIP diet can provide you with valuable support, tips, and encouragement along the way. You can find online forums, social media groups, or local meetups to connect with others.

6. **Focus on the Positive:** Instead of thinking about all the foods you can't eat, focus on the delicious and nourishing foods you can enjoy on the AIP diet. Shift your mindset from deprivation to abundance.

7. **Listen to Your Body:** Pay attention to how your body responds to different foods and adjust your diet accordingly. The AIP diet is not one-size-fits-all, so it's important to tailor it to your individual needs and preferences.

Remember, the AIP diet is not just about what you eat, but also about how you nourish your body and mind. Stay positive, stay committed, and most importantly, be kind to yourself as you embark on this journey towards better health and well-being.

Common Misconceptions about the AIP Diet.

Despite its proven benefits, there are some common misconceptions about the AIP diet that may prevent people from trying it or sticking to it. Let's address some of these misconceptions:

Misconception 1: The AIP Diet is Too Restrictive.

While the AIP diet does eliminate several food groups, it is not meant to be a lifelong restriction. The elimination phase is usually temporary, and foods are gradually reintroduced to identify individual triggers. Moreover, there are numerous delicious and satisfying foods that are AIP-friendly, allowing for a varied and enjoyable diet.

Misconception 2: The AIP Diet is Only for Extreme Cases.

While the AIP diet can be incredibly beneficial for individuals with severe autoimmune diseases, it can also benefit those with mild to moderate symptoms. Many people find that even minor changes in their diet can lead to significant improvements in their health and well-being.

Misconception 3: The AIP Diet is Expensive and Time-Consuming.

While it's true that the AIP diet may require some adjustments to your shopping and meal preparation routines, it doesn't have to be expensive or time-consuming. With proper planning and budgeting, you can follow the AIP diet without breaking the bank or spending hours in the kitchen.

Misconception 4: The AIP Diet is Just another Fad Diet.

The AIP diet is based on solid scientific principles and has been shown to be effective in managing autoimmune diseases. Unlike fad diets that promise quick fixes, the AIP diet focuses on long-term health and well-being through sustainable dietary changes.

Misconception 5: The AIP Diet Doesn't Allow for Enough Variety.

While the AIP diet does eliminate certain foods, there is still plenty of room for variety and creativity in your meals. By exploring new ingredients and cooking methods, you can discover a whole new world of delicious and nutritious foods that are AIP-friendly.

Misconception 6: The AIP Diet is a Cure-All.

While the AIP diet can significantly improve symptoms for many individuals with autoimmune diseases, it is not a cure-all. It is one part of a comprehensive approach to managing autoimmune conditions, which may also include medication, lifestyle changes, and other treatments as recommended by healthcare professionals.

Misconception 7: The AIP Diet is Too Difficult to Follow Long-Term.

While the elimination phase of the AIP diet may be challenging for some, many people find that they can successfully re-introduce foods and maintain a modified version of the AIP diet long-term. With proper planning, support, and a positive attitude, following the AIP diet can become a sustainable and rewarding lifestyle choice.

Misconception 8: The AIP Diet is Not Backed by Science.

Some critics argue that the AIP diet lacks scientific evidence to support its effectiveness. However, research has shown that the AIP diet can reduce inflammation, improve symptoms, and enhance quality of life for individuals with autoimmune diseases. While more research is needed, the existing evidence suggests that the AIP diet is a valid dietary approach for managing autoimmune conditions.

In conclusion, the AIP diet is a powerful tool for managing autoimmune diseases and improving overall health and well-being. By understanding the principles behind the AIP diet and dispelling common misconceptions, you can feel confident in your decision to embark on this transformative dietary journey.

Potential Challenges and How to Overcome Them.

1. **Social Pressure:** One of the biggest challenges of following the AIP Diet is social pressure. You may find it difficult to explain your dietary restrictions to friends and family or feel left out at social gatherings. To overcome this, it's important to communicate your needs clearly and assertively. Educate your loved ones about the reasons behind your dietary choices and

suggest alternative ways to socialize that don't revolve around food, such as going for a walk or attending a movie together.

2. **Cravings:** Eliminating certain foods from your diet can lead to cravings, especially during the initial phase of the AIP Diet. To overcome cravings, focus on incorporating a variety of flavors and textures into your meals. Experiment with new recipes and flavors to keep your meals exciting and satisfying. Additionally, make sure you're eating enough nutrient-dense foods to prevent feelings of deprivation.

3. **Meal Planning and Preparation:** Following the AIP Diet requires careful meal planning and preparation, which can be challenging for some people, especially those with busy schedules. To overcome this challenge, set aside time each week to plan your meals and prepare ingredients in advance. Invest in kitchen tools and appliances that make meal prep easier, such as a slow cooker or food processor. You can also consider batch cooking and freezing meals for later use.

4. **Expense:** Some people may find that following the AIP Diet is more expensive than their previous diet, as it often requires purchasing higher-quality, organic, and grass-fed ingredients. To overcome this challenge, prioritize your purchases by focusing on the most nutrient-dense foods and buying in bulk when possible. You can also look for sales and discounts or consider growing your own vegetables and herbs to reduce costs.

5. **Emotional Eating:** Many people use food as a coping mechanism for stress, boredom, or other emotions. The AIP Diet may challenge your relationship with food and require you

to find alternative ways to cope with emotions. To overcome emotional eating, practice mindful eating, and pay attention to your body's hunger and fullness cues. Find other ways to manage stress and emotions, such as meditation, yoga, or journaling.

6. **Travel and Dining Out:** Traveling and dining out can be challenging while following the AIP Diet, as you may have limited options or be unsure of the ingredients used in restaurant meals. To overcome this challenge, plan ahead by researching restaurants that offer AIP-friendly options or bring your own snacks and meals when traveling. Communicate your dietary needs to restaurant staff and ask questions about how dishes are prepared.

By being aware of these potential challenges and having strategies in place to overcome them, you can successfully navigate the AIP Diet and experience its many benefits. Remember, it's okay to have setbacks and challenges along the way. What's important is your commitment to your health and well-being, and your willingness to adapt and find solutions that work for you.

PREPARING YOUR KITCHEN.

Setting up your kitchen for success is essential when starting the AIP diet. Here are some tips to help you prepare:

1. **Clear out Non-AIP Foods:** Go through your pantry, refrigerator, and freezer, and remove any foods that are not AIP-compliant. This includes grains, legumes, dairy products, processed foods, and anything else on the list of foods to avoid.

2. **Stock Up on AIP-Friendly Foods:** Make sure you have plenty of AIP-friendly foods on hand, including vegetables, fruits, quality meats, fish and shellfish, healthy fats, fermented foods, bone broth, and herbal teas. Consider shopping at local farmers' markets or health food stores for the freshest options.

3. **Invest in Quality Kitchen Tools:** Having the right kitchen tools can make preparing AIP meals much easier and more enjoyable. Some essential tools to consider include a good quality chef's knife, cutting board, vegetable peeler, blender or food processor, and a set of cooking pots and pans.

4. **Organize Your Kitchen:** Arrange your kitchen in a way that makes cooking on the AIP diet convenient and efficient. Keep AIP-friendly foods in easy-to-reach places and store them in clear containers for quick identification.

5. **Plan Your Meals:** Meal planning is key to success on the AIP diet. Take some time each week to plan your meals, make a shopping list, and prep ingredients in advance. This will help you stay on track and avoid last-minute temptations.

6. **Batch Cooking:** Consider batch cooking large quantities of AIP-friendly meals and freezing them for later use. This can save you time and effort on busy days when you don't feel like cooking from scratch.

7. **Label Foods Clearly:** If you live with others who are not following the AIP diet, make sure to clearly label AIP-friendly foods to avoid confusion.

Essential Kitchen Tools for Cooking on the AIP Diet.

Having the right kitchen tools can make cooking on the AIP diet much easier and more enjoyable. Here are some essential tools to consider:

1. **Chef's Knife:** A good quality chef's knife is essential for chopping vegetables, fruits, and meats.

2. **Cutting Board:** A sturdy cutting board is necessary for preparing ingredients safely and efficiently.

3. **Vegetable Peeler:** A vegetable peeler is useful for peeling vegetables and fruits.

4. **Blender or Food Processor:** A blender or food processor can be used to puree soups, sauces, and smoothies.

5. **Cooking Pots and Pans:** A set of high-quality cooking pots and pans is essential for preparing AIP meals.

6. **Slow Cooker or Instant Pot:** A slow cooker or Instant Pot can make meal preparation easier, especially on busy days.

7. **Storage Containers:** Invest in a set of storage containers for storing leftovers and prepped ingredients.

Meal Planning and Batch Cooking on the AIP Diet.

Meal planning and batch cooking can save you time and effort on the AIP diet. Here are some tips to help you get started:

1. **Plan Your Meals:** Take some time each week to plan your meals, make a shopping list, and prep ingredients in advance.

2. **Batch Cooking:** Consider batch cooking large quantities of AIP-friendly meals and freezing them for later use. This can save you time and effort on busy days.

3. **Use Leftovers Wisely:** Repurpose leftovers into new meals to reduce waste and save time.

4. **Stay Flexible:** Don't be afraid to change your meal plans based on what's available and what you're in the mood for.

By preparing your kitchen and equipping yourself with the right tools and mindset, you can set yourself up for success on the AIP diet. Remember, it's not just about what you eat, but also how you nourish your body and mind. Stay positive, stay

committed, and most importantly, be kind to yourself as you
embark on this journey towards better health and well-being.

TROUBLESHOOTING AND COMMON QUESTIONS.

Following the Autoimmune Protocol (AIP) diet can be life-changing for many people, but it is not without challenges. Let's go over some common challenges on the AIP diet and provide practical strategies to overcome them.

Common Challenges on the AIP Diet.

1. **Social Isolation:** One of the most challenging aspects of the AIP diet is feeling isolated or left out in social situations where food plays an important role. It can be a challenge to find AIP-compliant meals at restaurants and events.

2. **Food Boredom:** Another common difficulty is becoming bored with the AIP diet's restricted meal alternatives. Eating the same foods every day might cause food fatigue and make it harder to stick to the diet over time.

3. **Cravings:** Cravings for non-compliant foods can be intense, particularly in the early stages of the AIP. This can make it difficult to stay on course and resist temptation.

4. **Nutrient Deficiencies:** The AIP diet eliminates many foods that are rich in certain nutrients, such as dairy and wheat. Without careful planning, it is possible to become deficient in essential nutrients such as calcium, vitamin D, and magnesium.

5. **Lack of Support:** If you don't have support from friends, family, or healthcare providers, sticking to the AIP diet can be difficult. Without support and understanding, it's easy to get discouraged and give up.

Strategies to Overcome Common Challenges.

1. **Plan Ahead:** Planning is essential for overcoming many of the challenges of the AIP diet. Plan your meals ahead of time, look up restaurant menus, and bring along AIP-friendly snacks when you go out.

2. **Be Creative in the Kitchen:** Try out new recipes and ingredients to keep your meals exciting and varied. Look online or in AIP cookbooks for new and delicious meal ideas.

3. **Find Support:** Joining a support group or online community of AIP dieters can provide you with the encouragement and support you need to stay motivated. Share your experiences, seek advice, and celebrate your achievements with people who understand what you're going through.

4. **Focus on the Benefits:** Remind yourself why you began the AIP diet in the first place. Whether you're trying to improve your health, reduce inflammation, or manage a chronic condition, focusing on the benefits helps keep you motivated and dedicated.

5. **Practice Mindfulness:** Mindful eating can help you stay present and enjoy your food more, reducing your chances of

feeling deprived or unsatisfied. Take your time to savor each bite, and pay attention to how different foods make you feel.

6. **Seek Professional Guidance:** If you're having difficulty sticking to the AIP diet, consider consulting with a healthcare professional or nutritionist who is conversant with the protocol. They can provide you personalized advice and support to help you succeed.

By recognizing and addressing these common challenges, you can overcome obstacles on the AIP diet and experience the many benefits it provides. With determination, planning, and support, you may successfully navigate the AIP diet while improving your health and well-being.

FAQs and Answers.

We'll address 13 frequently asked questions (FAQs) concerning the Autoimmune Protocol (AIP) diet to help you navigate common obstacles and uncertainties.

1. What is the Autoimmune Protocol (AIP) Diet?

The AIP diet is a therapeutic eating approach that aims to reduce inflammation and heal the gut by eliminating potentially inflammatory foods and focusing on nutrient-dense, healing foods.

2. What foods are allowed on the AIP diet?

The AIP diet focuses on whole foods such vegetables, fruits, meat, fish, and healthy fats. It eliminates grains, legumes, dairy, refined sugars, processed foods, and some additives.

3. How long should I be on the AIP diet?

The duration of the AIP diet varies per individual. Some people may notice improvements in their symptoms after a few weeks, whilst others may need to follow the diet for several months to see meaningful results.

4. Can I reintroduce foods after following the AIP diet?

Yes, the AIP diet is meant to be a brief elimination diet. After a period of strict abstinence, gradually reintroduce foods to discover which ones may be causing problems.

5. Can I eat out while following the AIP diet?

Eating out can be challenging, but it is feasible with proper planning. Look for restaurants that provide AIP-friendly options, or call ahead to inquire about menu items.

6. Can I drink alcohol on the AIP diet?

Alcohol is generally not suggested on the AIP diet because it might cause inflammation and worsen symptoms. However, some people may tolerate small amounts of certain alcohols.

7. Are there any supplements recommended on the AIP diet?

While food is the best source of nutrition, some people may benefit from supplements like probiotics, fish oil, and vitamin D. Before taking any supplements, consult your doctor.

8. How can I control cravings while following the AIP diet?

Cravings can be controlled by eating nutrient-dense foods, staying hydrated, and finding alternative ways to cope with stress or emotional eating.

9. Can I follow the AIP diet if I am vegetarian or vegan?

Yes, you can follow a vegetarian or vegan variation of the AIP diet that focuses on plant-based proteins, vegetables, fruits, and healthy fats. It may be more challenging to meet nutrient needs without animal products.

10. How do I stay motivated on the AIP diet?

Staying motivated on the AIP diet can be challenging, but focusing on your health goals, tracking your progress, as well as receiving encouragement from others will help keep you going.

11. Can I exercise while on the AIP diet?

Yes, moderate exercise is generally safe and recommended while on the AIP diet. However, listen to your body and adjust your activity level as necessary.

12. Will the AIP diet help me lose weight?

Weight loss can occur as a result of following the AIP diet, especially if you are eliminating processed foods in substitution for whole, nutrient-dense foods. Weight loss, should however, not be the primary goal of the AIP Diet.

13. Can children follow the AIP diet?

Children can follow a modified version of the AIP diet under the supervision of a healthcare professional or nutritionist. It is important to ensure that they are getting all of the nutrients required for growth and development.

In a nutshell, the AIP diet can be a powerful tool for improving your health and managing autoimmune conditions. By following these tips and guidelines, you can confidently manage the challenges of the AIP diet and achieve your health goals.

Tips for Eating Out and Socializing on the AIP Diet.

Eating out and socializing can be challenging when following the Autoimmune Protocol (AIP) diet, but with some planning and preparation, you can enjoy these experiences while adhering to your dietary needs. This chapter will provide you with practical tips and strategies for managing restaurants and social gatherings while on the AIP diet.

1. **Research and Plan Ahead:** Before going out to eat, research restaurants in your area that provide AIP-friendly options or are willing to accommodate your dietary needs. Look up menus online or call ahead to learn about menu items and preparation methods.

2. **Communicate Your Dietary Needs:** When dining out, don't be afraid to inform the restaurant staff about your dietary restrictions. Ask questions about ingredients, cooking methods, and substitutes to ensure that the meal meets your dietary requirements.

3. **Be Prepared with Snacks:** It is always a good idea to bring AIP-friendly snacks with you whether socializing or traveling. This way, if there are only a few food options available, you'll have a healthy alternative to choose from.

4. **Focus on Whole Foods:** When eating out, choose basic dishes prepared with whole, unprocessed ingredients. Avoid heavily seasoned foods and sauces, as these may contain non-compliant ingredients.

5. **Customize Your Order:** Many restaurants are willing to accommodate dietary restrictions and can customize dishes to match your specific needs. Don't be afraid to request substitutes or tweaks to make a dish AIP-friendly.

6. **Look for Hidden Ingredients:** Be cautious of hidden ingredients that may not be obvious. Sauces, marinades, and dressings, for example, may contain ingredients such as soy, gluten, or dairy that are not compliant.

7. **Avoid Cross-Contamination:** Cross-contamination can occur when food is prepared on surfaces or using utensils that have been in contact with non-compliant ingredients. When dining out, ask about the restaurant's practices to prevent cross-contamination.

8. **Choose Restaurants Carefully:** Some restaurants are more AIP-friendly than others. For example, farm-to-table restaurants, Mediterranean restaurants, and steakhouses can often have alternatives that can be easily modified to fit the AIP diet.

9. **Be Mindful of Alcohol:** Alcohol is often prohibited on the AIP diet as it can be inflammatory. If you choose to drink

alcohol, opt for AIP-friendly options such dry wines or hard cider produced from 100% fruit juice.

10. **Practice Mindful Eating:** When socializing, focus on enjoying the company of people over the food. Practice mindful eating by savoring each bite and paying attention to your body's signs for hunger and fullness.

By following these guidelines, you can navigate restaurants and social occasions with confidence while adhering to the AIP diet. With a little planning and preparation, you can enjoy tasty meals and meaningful social interactions without compromising your health goals.

Tips for Communicating Your Dietary Needs to Others.

1. **Be Clear and Specific:** When communicating your dietary needs to others, be explicit about what you can and cannot eat. Give examples of foods that are acceptable on the AIP diet and those that should be avoided.

2. **Educate others on the AIP Diet:** Many people are unfamiliar with the AIP diet and may not comprehend your dietary restrictions. Take the time to educate others about the AIP diet and why it is beneficial to your health.

3. **Use Positive Language:** When discussing your dietary needs, avoid sounding restrictive or negative. Instead of saying, "I can't eat that," say, "I choose to eat foods that support my health."

4. **Be Assertive:** Do not be scared to assertively state your dietary needs. It's critical to advocate for yourself and ensure that your nutritional needs are met.

5. **Provide Alternatives:** When attending social gatherings or events where food is served, offer to bring an AIP-compliant meal. This way, you'll have a safe alternative to enjoy, and others can try AIP-friendly foods.

6. **Ask for Support:** If you're going out to eat with friends or family, ask for their help in finding an AIP-friendly restaurant. Explain why sticking to the AIP diet is so important to you.

7. **Be Flexible:** While adhering to the AIP diet is essential, it is also necessary to be flexible and open to explore new foods and experiences. Look for creative ways to enjoy social gatherings without compromising your dietary needs.

8. **Express Gratitude:** When people meet your dietary requirements, show gratitude and appreciation. Let them know that you appreciate their support and understanding.

9. **Set Boundaries:** If others pressure you to eat foods that are not AIP-compliant, it is important to set boundaries and politely decline. Remember, your health comes first.

10. **Lead by Example:** By following the AIP diet and prioritizing your health, you can motivate others to make healthier choices as well. Lead by example and show others that eating healthy can be delicious and enjoyable.

By following these tips for communicating your dietary needs to others, you can confidently navigate social situations while staying compliant to the AIP diet. With a little planning and preparation, you can enjoy meaningful social interactions without compromising your health goals.

AIP BREAKFAST RECIPES.

SWEET POTATO BREAKFAST BOWL.

Preparation Time: 10 minutes

Cooking Time: 20 minutes

Ingredients:

- 1 medium sweet potato, peeled and cubed
- 1 tablespoon coconut oil
- 1/2 teaspoon cinnamon
- 1/4 cup coconut milk
- 1 tablespoon maple syrup (optional)
- 1/4 cup chopped nuts or seeds (optional)

Directions:

- Steam or boil sweet potato cubes until tender, about 15-20 minutes.
- In a skillet, heat coconut oil over medium heat.
- Add cooked sweet potato cubes and cinnamon. Cook for 2-3 minutes, stirring occasionally.
- Stir in coconut milk and maple syrup, if using. Cook for an additional minute.
- Transfer to a bowl and top with chopped nuts or seeds, if desired.

Serving Method:

Serve warm.

COCONUT FLOUR PORRIDGE.

Preparation Time: 5 minutes

Cooking Time: 5 minutes

Ingredients:

- 1/4 cup coconut flour
- 1 cup coconut milk
- 1/2 teaspoon cinnamon
- 1/4 teaspoon vanilla extract
- 1 tablespoon maple syrup (optional)

Directions:

- In a small saucepan, whisk together coconut flour, coconut milk, cinnamon, and vanilla extract.
- Cook over medium heat, stirring constantly, until thickened, about 3-5 minutes.
- Stir in maple syrup, if using.

Serving Method:

Serve warm.

AIP BREAKFAST SAUSAGE.

Preparation Time: 10 minutes

Cooking Time: 10 minutes

Ingredients:

- 1 pound ground pork
- 1 teaspoon dried sage

- 1/2 teaspoon garlic powder
- 1/2 teaspoon onion powder
- 1/2 teaspoon salt
- 1/4 teaspoon ground black pepper (omit for AIP)
- 1 tablespoon coconut oil (for cooking)

Directions:

- In a bowl, combine ground pork, sage, garlic powder, onion powder, salt, and pepper.
- Mold the mixture into small patties.
- In a skillet, heat the coconut oil over medium heat.
- Cook patties for 3-4 minutes per side, or until cooked through.

Serving Method:

Serve hot.

PLANTAIN WAFFLES.

Preparation Time: 10 minutes

Cooking Time: 10 minutes

Ingredients:

- 2 ripe plantains
- 2 eggs
- 2 tablespoons coconut oil, melted
- 1/2 teaspoon cinnamon
- 1/4 teaspoon salt

Directions:

- Preheat waffle iron and grease with coconut oil.
- Peel plantains and place them in a blender or food processor.
- Add eggs, coconut oil, cinnamon, and salt. Blend until smooth.
- Pour batter onto the preheated waffle iron and cook according to the manufacturer's instructions.

Serving Method:

Serve warm.

TURMERIC GINGER SMOOTHIE.

Preparation Time: 5 minutes

Cooking Time: 0 minutes

Ingredients:

- 1 cup coconut milk
- 1 banana
- 1/2 inch fresh ginger, peeled
- 1/2 teaspoon ground turmeric
- 1/2 teaspoon ground cinnamon
- 1 tablespoon honey (optional)

Directions:

- In a blender, combine coconut milk, banana, ginger, turmeric, cinnamon, and honey.
- Blend until smooth.

Serving Method:

Serve cold.

APPLE CINNAMON PORRIDGE.

Prep time: 5 minutes

Cooking time: 10 minutes

Ingredients:

- -1/2 cup coconut milk
- Add 1/2 cup water and 1/2 cup shredded apple.
- Use 1/4 cup coconut flour and 1/2 teaspoon cinnamon.
- 1/4 teaspoon nutmeg.
- one tablespoon maple syrup (optional)

Directions:

- Heat coconut milk and water in a small saucepan till simmering.
- Stir in the shredded apple, coconut flour, cinnamon, nutmeg, and maple syrup (if using).
- Cook over low heat, stirring constantly, until thickened, about 5-7 minutes.

Serving Method:

Serve warm.

BLUEBERRY COCONUT SMOOTHIE.

Preparation Time: 5 minutes

Cooking Time: 0 minutes

Ingredients:

- 1 cup coconut milk and 1/2 cup frozen blueberries.
- One-half banana
- One tablespoon of coconut butter
- Ingredients: - 1/2 teaspoon vanilla extract

Directions:

- In a blender, combine the coconut milk, blueberries, banana, coconut butter, and vanilla extract.
- Blend until smooth.

Serving Method:

Serve chilled.

CARROT CAKE BREAKFAST COOKIES.

Prep Time: 10 minutes

Cooking Time: 15 minutes

Ingredients:

- 1 cup shredded carrots
- 1/2 cup coconut flour
- 1/2 cup shredded coconut.
- 1/4 cup melted coconut oil
- 1/4 cup maple syrup.
- 1 teaspoon of cinnamon.
- 1/2 teaspoon ginger

Directions:

- Preheat the oven to 350°F/175°C, and prepare a baking sheet with parchment paper.
- In a large mixing bowl, combine the carrots, coconut flour, shredded coconut, coconut oil, maple syrup, cinnamon, ginger, and nutmeg.
- Mix until thoroughly blended.
- Shape the mixture into cookies and place on the prepared baking sheet.
- Bake for 12–15 minutes, or until golden brown.

Serving Method:

Serve warm or room temperature.

PUMPKIN PIE SMOOTHIE.

Prep Time: 5 minutes

Cooking Time: 0 minutes

Ingredients:

- Use 1/2 cup pumpkin puree
- 1/2 banana
- 1 cup coconut milk.
- 1/2 teaspoon cinnamon
- 1/4 teaspoon nutmeg.
- 1/4 teaspoon ginger
- 1 tablespoon maple syrup (optional)

Directions:

- In a blender, combine the pumpkin puree, banana, coconut milk, cinnamon, nutmeg, ginger, and maple syrup, if desired.
- Blend until smooth.

Serving Method:

Serve chilled.

TIGER NUT FLOUR PANCAKES.

Prep Time: 10 minutes

Cooking Time: 10 minutes

Ingredients:

- -1 cup tiger nut flour
- 1/2 teaspoon baking soda.
- 2 eggs
- -1/2 cup coconut milk
- 1 tablespoon heated coconut oil

Directions:

- In a bowl, whisk together, the tiger nut flour and baking soda.
- In a separate bowl, beat the eggs, then stir the coconut milk and melted coconut oil.
- Pour wet and dry ingredients together and mix thoroughly.
- Heat a greased skillet over medium heat.
- Pour batter onto the skillet to form pancakes.
- Cook each side for 2-3 minutes, or until golden brown.

Serving Method:

Serve warm.

BERRY CHIA SEED PUDDING.

Preparation Time: 5 minutes (plus overnight chilling)

Cooking Time: 0 minutes

Ingredients:

- 1/4 cup chia seeds.
- 1 cup coconut milk.
- Add 1/2 teaspoon vanilla extract
- 1 tablespoon maple syrup (optional)
- Mixed berries, for toppings

Directions:

- In a bowl, mix chia seeds, coconut milk, vanilla extract, and maple syrup (if using).
- Cover and refrigerate overnight, or for at least 4 hours, until thickened.
- Before serving, stir well and top with mixed berries.

PUMPKIN SPICE MUFFINS.

Prep Time: 10 minutes

Cooking Time: 20 minutes

Ingredients:

- 1 cup pumpkin puree
- 1/4 cup melted coconut oil
- 1/4 cup maple syrup
- 2 eggs
- Use 1/2 cup coconut flour and 1 teaspoon baking soda
- 1 teaspoon of cinnamon.
- -1/2 teaspoon ginger
- 1/4 teaspoon nutmeg

Directions:

- Preheat the oven to 350°F/175°C and line a muffin tin with paper liners.
- In a bowl, mix pumpkin puree, coconut oil, maple syrup, and eggs.
- Add coconut flour, baking soda, cinnamon, ginger, and nutmeg. Mix until well blended.
- Scoop the batter into muffin cups.
- Bake for 20 to 25 minutes, or until when a toothpick put in the center comes out clean.
- Allow to cool before serving.

GREEN BANANA FLOUR PANCAKES.

Prep Time: 10 minutes

Cooking Time: 10 minutes

Ingredients:

- Use 1 cup of green banana flour and 2 eggs
- -1/2 cup coconut milk
- One-half teaspoon baking soda

- 1/2 teaspoon cinnamon
- 1/4 teaspoon of salt

Directions:

- In a bowl, whisk together green banana flour, eggs, the milk from the coconuts, baking soda, cinnamon, and salt.
- Preheat a skillet that has been greased over medium heat.
- Pour batter into the skillet in order to form pancakes.
- Cook each side for 2-3 minutes, or until golden brown.

Serving Method:

Serve warm.

MANGO COCONUT SMOOTHIE.

Prep Time: 5 minutes

Cooking Time: 0 minutes

Ingredients:

- 1 cup coconut milk
- 1/2 cup frozen mango chunks.
- One-half banana
- 1 tablespoon of shredded coconut

Directions:

- In a blender, pour coconut milk, mango chunks, banana, and shredded coconut.
- Blend until smooth.

Serving Method:

Serve chilled.

CINNAMON RAISIN BREAKFAST COOKIES.

Prep Time: 10 minutes

Cooking Time: 15 minutes

Ingredients:

- Use 1/2 cup coconut flour and 1/2 teaspoon baking soda.
- -1/2 teaspoon cinnamon
- A pinch of salt
- 1/4 cup melted coconut oil
- 1/4 cup maple syrup
- Add 1 egg and 1/4 cup raisins

Directions:

- Set the oven to 350°F/175°C and line a baking sheet with parchment paper.
- In a bowl, combine coconut flour, baking soda, cinnamon, and salt.
- In a separate bowl, mix melted coconut oil, maple syrup, and egg.
- Add the wet and dry ingredients, then fold in raisins.
- Form the dough into cookies and place on the prepared baking sheet.
- Bake for 12–15 minutes, or until it turns golden brown.
- Allow to cool before serving.

AIP LUNCH AND DINNER RECIPES.

AIP CHICKEN SALAD.

Prep Time: 15 minutes

Cooking Time: 20 minutes (for chicken)

Ingredients:

- 2 boneless, skinless chicken breasts
- 1 avocado, mashed
- ¼ cup chopped fresh cilantro
- ¼ cup chopped green onions
- ¼ diced cucumber
- ¼ cup diced red bell pepper
- Juice of one lime
- Salt and pepper to taste

Directions:

- Preheat your oven over 375°F (190°C)
- Season the chicken breasts with salt and pepper, then place them on a baking sheet lined with parchment paper.
- Bake the chicken breasts for about 20 minutes, or until they are cooked through and no longer sink in the center. Let them cook slightly and, then chop them into bite-sized pieces.

- In a large bowl, combine the chopped chicken, mashed avocado. Cilantro, green onions, cucumber, red bell pepper, and lime juice. Mix until well combined.
- Season the chicken salad with additional salt and pepper to taste, if needed.

Serving Method:

Serve the AIP chicken salad immediately, or refrigerate for later.

Note: It can be enjoyed on its own, served on top of salad greens, wrapped in lettuce leaves, or stuffed into a gluten-free wrap for a delicious and satisfying meal.

BUTTERNUT SQUASH SOUP.

Prep Time: 15 minutes

Cooking Time: 30 minutes

Ingredients:

- 1 medium butternut squash, peeled, seeded, and sliced.
- 1 onion, chopped
- 2 cloves garlic, minced
- 4 cups chicken or vegetable broth
- 1/2 teaspoon ground ginger
- 1/2 teaspoon ground cinnamon
- Salt, to taste
- Coconut milk (optional, for garnish)

Directions:

- In a sizeable pot, sauté onion and garlic until softened.

- Add butternut squash, broth, ginger, cinnamon, and salt.
  Bring to a boil, then reduce heat and simmer for 20-25
  minutes, or until squash is tender.
- Blend soup until smooth using an immersion blender or
  regular blender.

Serving Method:

Serve hot, garnished with a swirl of coconut milk if desired.

ZUCCHINI NOODLES WITH PESTO.

Preparation Time: 15 minutes

Cooking Time: 5 minutes

Ingredients:

- 2 large zucchinis, spiralized into noodles
- 1/2 cup fresh basil leaves
- 1/4 cup pine nuts
- 1/4 cup olive oil
- 1 clove garlic, minced
- Salt, to taste

Directions:

- In a food processor, blend basil, pine nuts, olive oil,
  garlic, and salt until smooth.
- In a skillet over medium heat, sauté zucchini noodles for
  3-5 minutes, or until tender.
- Toss cooked zucchini noodles with pesto.

Serving Method:

Serve hot.

ROASTED CARROT AND PARSNIP SOUP.

Prep Time: 15 minutes

Cooking Time: 30 minutes

Ingredients:

- 4 carrots, peeled and chopped
- 2 parsnips, peeled and chopped
- 1 onion, chopped
- 2 cloves garlic, minced
- 4 cups chicken or vegetable broth
- 1/2 teaspoon ground cumin
- 1/2 teaspoon ground coriander
- Salt, to taste

Directions:

- Preheat oven to 400°F (200°C).
- Place carrots, parsnips, onion, and garlic on a baking sheet. Simply roast for about 20 - 25 minutes or until the veggies are soft.
- In a large pot, combine roasted vegetables, broth, cumin, coriander, and salt. Bring to a boil, then lower the heat and allow to simmer for 5-10 minutes.
- Blend soup until smooth using an immersion blender or regular blender.

Serving Method:

Serve hot.

AIP CAESAR SALAD.

Prep Time: 15 minutes

Cooking Time: 0 minutes

Ingredients:

For the dressing:

- 1/2 cup coconut milk yogurt
- 2 tablespoons lemon juice
- 1 clove garlic, minced
- 2 anchovy fillets (optional)
- 1/4 cup olive oil
- Salt, to taste

For the salad:

- Romaine lettuce, chopped
- A handful of AIP-friendly bacon bits
- A handful of AIP-friendly croutons (optional)

Directions:

- In a blender, combine coconut milk yogurt, lemon juice, garlic, anchovy fillets (if using), olive oil, and salt. Blend until smooth.
- In a large bowl, toss romaine lettuce with dressing until well coated.
- Top with bacon bits and croutons, if using.

Serving Method:

Serve cold.

BAKED SALMON WITH LEMON AND DILL.

Prep Time: 10 minutes

Cooking Time: 15 minutes

Ingredients:

- 4 salmon fillets
- 2 tablespoons olive oil
- 1 tablespoon lemon juice
- 1 tablespoon chopped fresh dill
- Salt and pepper, to taste

Directions:

- Preheat oven to 375°F (190°C).
- Spread the salmon fillets on a baking sheet lined with parchment paper.
- In a small bowl, mix olive oil, lemon juice, dill, salt, and pepper.
- Apply the mixture to the salmon fillets.
- Bake for 12-15 minutes, or until salmon is cooked through and flakes easily with a fork.

Serving Method:

Serve hot.

CAULIFLOWER RICE STIR-FRY.

Prep Time: 10 minutes

Cooking Time: 10 minutes

Ingredients:

- 1 head cauliflower, grated into rice-like pieces
- 2 tablespoons coconut aminos
- 1 tablespoon coconut oil
- 1/2 onion, chopped
- 1 carrot, diced
- 1 bell pepper, diced
- 1 cup broccoli florets
- Salt, to taste

Directions:

- In a large skillet, heat coconut oil over medium heat.
- Add onion, carrot, bell pepper, and broccoli. Sauté for 5-7 minutes, or until vegetables are tender.
- Add cauliflower rice and coconut aminos. Cook for an additional 3-5 minutes, stirring frequently.
- Season with salt to taste.

Serving Method:

Serve hot.

SWEET POTATO AND APPLE SOUP.

Prep Time: 15 minutes

Cooking Time: 30 minutes

Ingredients:

- 2 sweet potatoes, peeled and chopped
- 2 apples, peeled, cored, and chopped
- 1 onion, chopped

- 4 cups chicken or vegetable broth
- 1/2 teaspoon ground cinnamon
- 1/2 teaspoon ground nutmeg
- Salt, to taste

Directions:

- In a large pot, combine sweet potatoes, apples, onion, broth, cinnamon, nutmeg, and salt. Bring to a boil, then reduce heat and simmer for 20-25 minutes, or until the veggies are soft.
- Blend soup until smooth using an immersion blender or regular blender.

Serving Method:

Serve hot.

AIP COLESLAW.

Preparation Time: 10 minutes

Cooking Time: 0 minutes

Ingredients:

- 1/2 head green cabbage, thinly sliced
- 1/2 head purple cabbage, thinly sliced
- 2 carrots, grated
- 1/2 cup coconut milk yogurt
- 2 tablespoons apple cider vinegar
- 1 tablespoon honey (optional)
- Salt, to taste

Directions:

- In a large bowl, combine green cabbage, purple cabbage, and carrots.
- In a small bowl, mix coconut milk yogurt, apple cider vinegar, honey (if using), and salt until well combined.
- Pour the dressing over the cabbage mixture and toss until evenly coated.

Serving Method:

Serve chilled.

TURKEY MEATBALLS WITH ZUCCHINI NOODLES.

Preparation Time: 15 minutes

Cooking Time: 25 minutes

Ingredients:

- 1 pound ground turkey
- 1/4 cup coconut flour
- 1/4 cup coconut milk
- 1/2 teaspoon garlic powder
- 1/2 teaspoon onion powder
- Salt, to taste
- 2 large zucchinis, spiralized into noodles

Directions:

- Preheat oven to 400°F (200°C) and line a baking sheet with parchment paper.

- In a bowl, mix together ground turkey, coconut flour, coconut milk, garlic powder, onion powder, and salt until well combined.
- Shape the mixture into meatballs and place them on the prepared baking sheet.
- Bake for 20-25 minutes, or until cooked through.
- In a skillet over medium heat, sauté zucchini noodles for 3-5 minutes, or until tender.

Serving Method:

Serve meatballs over zucchini noodles.

ROASTED BRUSSELS SPROUTS WITH BACON.

Preparation Time: 10 minutes

Cooking Time: 25 minutes

Ingredients:

- 1 pound Brussels sprouts, trimmed and cut into half
- 4 slices AIP-friendly bacon, chopped
- 2 tablespoons olive oil
- Salt and pepper, to taste

Directions:

- Preheat oven to 400°F (200°C) and line a baking sheet with parchment paper.
- In a mixing bowl, toss Brussels sprouts with olive oil, salt, and pepper.
- 3. Spread Brussels sprouts on the prepared baking sheet and scatter chopped bacon on top.

- 4. Roast for 20-25 minutes, or until Brussels sprouts are tender and bacon is crispy.

Serving Method:

Serve hot.

BEEF AND VEGETABLE STIR-FRY.

Prep Time: 15 minutes

Cooking Time: 15 minutes

Ingredients:

- 1 pound of beef sirloin, cut into thin slices
- 2 tablespoons coconut aminos
- 1 tablespoon coconut oil
- 1 onion, sliced
- 1 bell pepper, sliced
- 1 cup broccoli florets
- Salt and pepper, to taste

Directions:

- In a bowl, marinate beef slices in coconut aminos for 10 minutes.
- In a big skillet, heat the coconut oil over medium-high heat.
- Add onion, bell pepper, and broccoli. Sauté for 5-7 minutes, or until vegetables are tender.
- Add marinated beef to the skillet. Cook for an additional 5 minutes, or until beef is cooked through.
- Season with salt and pepper.

Serve hot.

AIP TUNA SALAD.

Prep Time: 10 minutes

Cooking Time: 0 minutes

Ingredients:

- 2 cans tuna, drained
- 1/2 cup coconut milk yogurt
- 1 tablespoon lemon juice
- 1/2 teaspoon garlic powder
- Salt and pepper, to taste
- Mixed greens, for serving

Directions:

- In a bowl, mix tuna, coconut milk yogurt, lemon juice, garlic powder, salt, and pepper until well combined.
- Serve tuna salad over mixed greens.

Serving Method:

Serve chilled.

CHICKEN AND VEGETABLE SKEWERS.

Prep Time: 20 minutes

Cooking Time: 15 minutes

Ingredients:

- 1 pound chicken breast, cut into cubes
- 1 zucchini, sliced
- 1 bell pepper, diced
- 1 onion, diced
- 2 tablespoons olive oil
- 1 tablespoon lemon juice
- 1 teaspoon dried oregano
- Salt and pepper, to taste

Directions:

- In a bowl, combine chicken cubes, zucchini, bell pepper, onion, olive oil, lemon juice, oregano, salt, and pepper. Marinate for 10 minutes.
- Thread marinated chicken and vegetables onto skewers.
- Grill skewers over medium heat for 10-15 minutes, or until chicken is cooked through.

Serving Method:

Serve hot.

CABBAGE AND APPLE SLAW.

Preparation Time: 10 minutes

Cooking Time: 0 minutes

Ingredients:

- 1/2 head green cabbage, thinly sliced
- 1 apple, julienned
- 1/4 cup coconut milk yogurt

- 1 tablespoon apple cider vinegar
- 1 teaspoon honey (optional)
- Salt, to taste

Directions:

- In a large bowl, combine green cabbage and apple.
- In a small bowl, mix coconut milk yogurt, apple cider vinegar, honey (if using), and salt until well combined.
- Pour the dressing over the cabbage and apple mixture and toss until well coated.

Serving Method:

Serve chilled.

LEMON HERB ROASTED CHICKEN.

Preparation Time: 10 minutes

Cooking Time: 1 hour

Ingredients:

- 1 full chicken (about 3-4 pounds)
- 1/4 cup olive oil
- 2 tablespoons lemon juice
- 2 cloves garlic, minced
- 1 tablespoon sliced fresh herbs (such as rosemary, thyme, or sage)
- Salt and pepper, to taste

Directions:

- Preheat oven to 375°F (190°C).

- In a small bowl, mix olive oil, lemon juice, garlic, herbs, salt, and pepper.
- Rub the mixture over the whole chicken, making sure to coat it evenly.
- Place the chicken in a roasting pan and roast for about 1 hour, or until the chicken reaches an internal temperature of 165°F (74°C).
- Let the chicken cool off for 10 minutes before carving.

Serving Method:

Serve hot.

AIP BROCCOLI SOUP.

Prep Time: 10 minutes

Cooking Time: 20 minutes

Ingredients:

- 1 head broccoli, chopped
- 1 onion, chopped
- 2 cloves garlic, minced
- 4 cups chicken or vegetable broth
- 1/2 cup coconut milk
- Salt, to taste

Directions:

- In a large pot, cook onion and garlic until softened.
- Add broccoli and broth. Bring to a boil, then reduce heat and simmer for 15-20 minutes, or until broccoli is tender.

- Blend soup until smooth using an immersion blender or regular blender.
- Stir in coconut milk and season with salt to taste.

Serving Method:

Serve hot.

ROASTED ROOT VEGETABLES.

Prep Time: 15 minutes

Cooking Time: 30 minutes

Ingredients:

- 2 carrots, peeled and chopped
- 2 parsnips, peeled and chopped
- 1 sweet potato, peeled and chopped
- 2 tablespoons olive oil
- Salt and pepper, to taste

Directions:

- Preheat oven to 400°F (200°C) and line a baking sheet with parchment paper.
- In a bowl, toss carrots, parsnips, and sweet potato with olive oil, salt, and pepper.
- Arrange the veggies in a single layer on the prepared baking sheet.
- Roast for 25-30 minutes, or until vegetables are tender and golden brown.

Serving Method:

Serve hot.

SHRIMP AND AVOCADO SALAD.

Prep Time: 15 minutes

Cooking Time: 5 minutes

Ingredients:

- 1 pound shrimp, peeled and cleaned
- 1 avocado, diced
- 1/2 red onion, thinly sliced
- 1/4 cup chopped fresh cilantro
- 2 tablespoons olive oil
- 1 tablespoon lemon juice
- Salt and pepper, to taste

Directions:

- In a skillet over medium heat, cook shrimp for 2-3 minutes per side, or until pink and cooked through.
- In a large bowl, combine cooked shrimp, avocado, red onion, and cilantro.
- In a small bowl, mix olive oil, lemon juice, salt, and pepper.
- Pour the dressing over the shrimp mixture and toss until well coated.

Serving Method:

Serve cold.

AIP SHEPHERD'S PIE.

Prep Time: 30 minutes

Cooking Time: 45 minutes

Ingredients:

For the filling:

- 1 pound ground beef
- 1 onion, chopped
- 2 carrots, diced
- 2 cloves garlic, minced
- 1 cup of beef or vegetable broth
- 1 teaspoon dried thyme
- Salt and pepper, to taste

For the topping:

- 2 pounds sweet potatoes, peeled and diced
- 2 tablespoons coconut oil
- Salt, to taste

Directions:

- Preheat oven to 375°F (190°C).
- In a skillet over medium heat, cook ground beef, onion, carrots, and garlic until beef is browned and vegetables are tender
- Add broth, thyme, salt, and pepper. Simmer for 10-15 minutes.
- Meanwhile, steam sweet potatoes until tender. Mash with coconut oil and salt.
- Spread the beef mixture in a baking dish.
- Top with mashed sweet potatoes.

- Bake for 20-25 minutes, or until the top is lightly browned.

Serving Method:

Serve hot.

AIP SNACKS AND APPETIZERS.

GUACAMOLE WITH VEGGIE STICKS.

Prep Time: 10 minutes

Cooking Time: 0 minutes

Ingredients:

- 2 ripe avocados
- 1 lime, juiced
- 1/4 cup chopped cilantro
- 1/4 cup diced red onion
- 1/2 teaspoon garlic powder
- Salt, to taste
- Assorted veggie sticks (carrots, celery, bell peppers)

Directions:

- In a bowl, smash the avocados with a fork.
- Add lime juice, chopped cilantro, diced red onion, garlic powder, and salt. Mix well.
- Serve with assorted veggie sticks.

Serving Method:

Serve chilled.

PLANTAIN CHIPS WITH AIP SALSA.

Prep Time: 10 minutes

Cooking Time: 15 minutes

Ingredients:

- 2 green plantains
- 2 tablespoons coconut oil, melted
- Salt, to taste

For the AIP salsa:

- 1/2 cup diced tomatoes
- 1/4 cup diced red onion
- 1/4 cup chopped cilantro
- 1 tablespoon lime juice
- Salt, to taste

Directions:

- Preheat the oven to 350°F/175°C and set a baking sheet with parchment paper.
- Peel and slice the plantains thinly.
- Mix the plantain slices, melted coconut oil, and salt.
- Arrange the plantain slices in a single layer on the prepped baking sheet.
- Bake for 15 minutes, or until golden brown and crispy.
- Meanwhile, prepare the AIP salsa by combining diced tomatoes, diced red onion, chopped cilantro, lime juice, and salt in a bowl.

Serving Method:

- Serve the plantain chips with the AIP salsa.

AIP TRAIL MIX (COCONUT FLAKES, DRIED FRUITS, SEEDS).

Preparation Time: 5 minutes

Cooking Time: 0 minutes

Ingredients:

- 1/2 cup coconut flakes
- 1/4 cup dried fruits (such as raisins, cranberries, chopped apricots)
- 1/4 cup mixed seeds (like pumpkin seeds and sunflower seeds)

Directions:

- Mix coconut flakes, dried fruits, and mixed seeds in a bowl.
- Store in an airtight container.

Serving Method:

Serve as a snack.

SWEET POTATO CHIPS.

Preparation Time: 10 minutes

Cooking Time: 25 minutes

Ingredients:

- 2 medium sweet potatoes, cut very thinly
- 2 tablespoons coconut oil, melted
- Salt, to taste

Directions:

- Preheat oven to 375°F (190°C) and line a baking sheet with parchment paper.
- In a bowl, toss sweet potato slices with melted coconut oil and salt.
- Spread the sweet potato slices in a single layer on the prepared baking sheet.
- Bake for 20-25 minutes, flipping halfway through, or until crispy.
- Let cool before serving.

Serving Method:

Serve as a snack.

CARROT STICKS WITH AIP RANCH DRESSING.

Preparation Time: 10 minutes

Cooking Time: 0 minutes

Ingredients:

- 4-5 carrots, peeled and cut into sticks

For the AIP ranch dressing:

- 1/2 cup coconut milk
- 2 tablespoons apple cider vinegar
- 1/2 teaspoon onion powder
- 1/2 teaspoon garlic powder
- 1/2 teaspoon dried dill

- Salt, to taste

Directions:

- In a bowl, mix coconut milk, apple cider vinegar, onion powder, garlic powder, dried dill, and salt until well combined.
- Serve carrot sticks with AIP ranch dressing for dipping.

Serving Method:

Serve carrot sticks with AIP ranch dressing for dipping.

COCONUT-CRUSTED CHICKEN TENDERS.

Prep Time: 15 minutes

Cooking Time: 20 minutes

Ingredients:

- 1 pound chicken tenders
- 1/2 cup coconut flour
- 2 eggs, beaten
- 1 cup shredded coconut
- Salt, to taste
- Coconut oil, for frying

Directions:

- Preheat oven to 400°F (200°C) and line a baking sheet with parchment paper.
- Season chicken tenders with salt.
- Dredge each chicken tender in coconut flour, dip in beaten eggs, coat with shredded coconut.

- Place the coated chicken tenders on the baking sheet that you've prepared.
- Bake for 15-20 minutes, or until chicken is cooked through and coconut is golden brown.

Serving Method:

Serve alongside your favorite dipping sauce.

AIP DEVILED EGGS.

Prep Time: 15 minutes

Cooking Time: 10 minutes

Ingredients:

- 6 hard-boiled eggs, peeled
- 2 tablespoons coconut milk
- 1 tablespoon apple cider vinegar
- 1/2 teaspoon mustard powder
- Salt, to taste
- Paprika (optional, for garnish)

Directions:

- Cut the hard-boiled eggs lengthwise into two and remove the yolks.
- In a bowl, mash the egg yolks with coconut milk, apple cider vinegar, mustard powder, and salt until smooth.
- Spoon the yolk mixture back into the egg whites.
- Sprinkle with paprika, if desired.

Serving Method:

Serve chilled.

BAKED SWEET POTATO FRIES.

Preparation Time: 15 minutes

Cooking Time: 25 minutes

Ingredients:

- 2 medium sweet potatoes, cut into fries
- 2 tablespoons coconut oil, melted
- Salt, to taste

Directions:

- Preheat oven to 425°F (220°C) and line a baking sheet with parchment paper.
- In a bowl, toss sweet potato fries with melted coconut oil and salt.
- Spread the sweet potato fries in a single layer on the prepared baking sheet.
- Bake for 20-25 minutes, flipping halfway through, or until crispy.
- Let cool slightly before serving.

Serving Method:

Serve warm.

AIP MEATBALLS.

Prep Time: 15 minutes

Cooking Time: 25 minutes

Ingredients:

- 1 pound ground beef
- 1/4 cup coconut flour
- 1/4 cup coconut milk
- 1/2 teaspoon garlic powder
- 1/2 teaspoon onion powder
- Salt, to taste

Directions:

- Preheat oven to 400°F (200°C) and line a baking sheet with parchment paper.
- In a bowl, mix together ground beef, coconut flour, coconut milk, garlic powder, onion powder, and salt until well combined.
- Mold the mixture into meatballs and place them on the prepped baking sheet.
- Bake for 20-25 minutes, or until cooked through.

Serving Method:

Serve with your favorite sauce.

CUCUMBER SLICES WITH AIP TZATZIKI SAUCE.

Prep Time: 15 minutes

Cooking Time: 0 minutes

Ingredients:

- 1 cucumber, sliced

For the AIP tzatziki sauce:

- 1/2 cup coconut milk yogurt
- 1/2 cucumber, shredded and squeezed to remove excess liquid
- 1 clove garlic, minced
- 1 tablespoon chopped fresh dill
- 1 tablespoon lemon juice
- Salt, to taste

Directions:

- In a bowl, mix coconut milk yogurt, grated cucumber, minced garlic, chopped fresh dill, lemon juice, and salt until well combined.
- Place the bowl in a refrigerator to chill while you prepare the cucumbers.
- Wash the cucumbers thoroughly and slice them thinly
- Arrange the cucumbers slices on a serving platter.
- Take the tzatziki sauce out of the refrigerator and give it a final stir.

Serving Method:

Serve cucumber slices with AIP tzatziki sauce for dipping.

BACON-WRAPPED DATES.

Prep Time: 15 minutes

Cooking Time: 15 minutes

Ingredients:

-   10 Medjool dates, pitted
-   5 slices of bacon, cut in half

Directions:

-   Preheat oven to 375°F (190°C) and line a baking sheet with parchment paper.
-   Stuff each date with a whole almond (optional).
-   Wrap each date with half a slice of bacon and secure with a toothpick.
-   Arrange the wrapped dates on the prepped baking sheet.
-   Bake for 12-15 minutes, or until the bacon is crispy.

Serving Method:

Serve warm as an appetizer.

AIP VEGGIE DIP (MADE WITH COCONUT YOGURT AND HERBS).

Prep Time: 10 minutes

Cooking Time: 0 minutes

Ingredients:

-   1 cup coconut milk yogurt
-   2 tablespoons chopped fresh herbs (such as parsley, chives, dill)
-   1 clove garlic, minced
-   Salt, to taste
-   Optional: squeeze of lemon juice for extra flavor

Directions:

- In a bowl, mix coconut milk yogurt, chopped fresh herbs, minced garlic, and salt until well combined.
- Mix well until all the ingredients are evenly distributed.
- Taste and adjust seasoning if necessary. If you'd like a tangier flavor, you can add a squeeze of lemon juice.
- Refrigerate for about 30 minutes to let the flavors meld together.

Serving Method:

Serve chilled with your favorite sliced vegetables such as carrots, cucumbers, bell peppers or celery.

COCONUT BACON.

Prep Time: 5 minutes

Cooking Time: 15 minutes

Ingredients:

- 1 cup coconut flakes
- 1 tablespoon coconut aminos
- 1/2 teaspoon smoked paprika
- 1/2 teaspoon garlic powder
- Salt, to taste

Directions:

- Preheat oven to 350°F (175°C) and set a baking sheet with parchment paper.
- In a bowl, mix coconut flakes, coconut aminos, smoked paprika, garlic powder, and salt until well combined.

- Spread the mixture in an even layer on the prepped baking sheet.
- Bake for 10-15 minutes, stirring occasionally, until crispy and golden brown.
- Let cool before serving.

Serving Method:

Serve as a topping for salads or snacks.

BAKED ZUCCHINI FRIES.

Prep Time: 15 minutes

Cooking Time: 20 minutes

Ingredients:

- 2 medium zucchinis, sliced into fries
- 1/4 cup coconut flour
- 2 eggs, beaten
- 1/2 cup shredded coconut
- Salt, to taste

Directions:

- Preheat oven to 425°F (220°C) and line a baking sheet with parchment paper.
- Dredge zucchini fries in coconut flour, dip in beaten eggs, coat with shredded coconut.
- Place the coated zucchini fries on the prepared baking sheet.
- Bake for 15-20 minutes, or until zucchini is tender and coating is crispy.

Serving Method:

Serve with your preferred dipping sauce.

AIP PIZZA BITES (USING A PLANTAIN BASE).

Prep Time: 15 minutes

Cooking Time: 20 minutes

Ingredients:

- 2 ripe plantains
- 1/4 cup coconut flour
- 2 tablespoons coconut oil, melted
- 1/2 teaspoon garlic powder
- 1/2 teaspoon onion powder
- Salt, to taste

AIP-friendly pizza sauce:

- Toppings of your choice (such as cooked chicken, bacon, vegetables)

Directions:

- Preheat oven to 375°F (190°C) and line a baking sheet with parchment paper.
- Peel and chop the plantains, then blend them in a food processor until smooth.
- Add coconut flour, melted coconut oil, garlic powder, onion powder, and salt to the plantain mixture. Blend until well combined.
- 4. Form the plantain dough into small rounds and place them on the prepared baking sheet.

- 5. Bake for 10 minutes.
- 6. Remove from the oven and top each plantain round with pizza sauce and toppings of your choice.
- Bake for an additional 10 minutes, or until toppings are heated through.

Serving Method:

Serve warm as a snack or appetizer.

APPLE SLICES WITH ALMOND BUTTER.

Prep Time: 5 minutes

Cooking Time: 0 minutes

Ingredients:

- 1 apple, sliced
- Almond butter, for dipping

Directions:

- Cut the apple into thin slices.
- Serve with almond butter to dip.
-

Serving Method:

Serve as a snack or light appetizer.

AIP AVOCADO BOATS (FILLED WITH TUNA OR CHICKEN SALAD).

Prep Time: 10 minutes

Cooking Time: 0 minutes

Ingredients:

-   2 avocados, halved and pitted

For the filling:

-   1 can tuna or cooked chicken, shredded
-   2 tablespoons coconut milk yogurt
-   1 tablespoon lemon juice
-   1/2 teaspoon garlic powder
-   Salt, to taste

Directions:

-   In a bowl, mix tuna or chicken with coconut milk yogurt, lemon juice, garlic powder, and salt until well combined.
-   Fill each avocado half with the tuna or chicken mixture.

Serving Method:

Serve as a light meal or snack.

ROASTED CAULIFLOWER BITES.

Prep Time: 10 minutes

Cooking Time: 25 minutes

Ingredients:

-   1 head cauliflower, diced into florets
-   2 tablespoons olive oil
-   1/2 teaspoon garlic powder

- Salt, to taste

Directions:

- Preheat oven to 425°F (220°C) and line a baking sheet with parchment paper.
- In a bowl, toss cauliflower florets with olive oil, garlic powder, and salt.
- Spread the cauliflower florets in a single layer on the prepared baking sheet.
- Roast for 20-25 minutes, or until cauliflower is tender and golden brown.

Serving Method:

Serve as an appetizer or side dish.

AIP ENERGY BALLS (MADE WITH DATES, COCONUT, AND SEEDS).

Preparation Time: 15 minutes

Cooking Time: 0 minutes

Ingredients:

- 1 cup pitted dates
- 1/2 cup shredded coconut
- 1/4 cup mixed seeds (like pumpkin seeds and sunflower seeds)
- 1/4 cup coconut oil, melted

Directions:

- In a food processor, blend dates, shredded coconut, mixed seeds, and melted coconut oil until a dough forms.
- Roll the dough into small balls.
- Refrigerate for at least 30 minutes before serving.

Serving Method:

Serve as a quick and energizing snack.

SMOKED SALMON CUCUMBER BITES.

Prep Time: 10 minutes

Cooking Time: 0 minutes

Ingredients:

- 1 cucumber, sliced
- Smoked salmon
- Fresh dill, for garnish

Directions:

- Slice the cucumber into thin rounds.
- Top each cucumber slice with a piece of smoked salmon.
- Garnish with fresh dill.

Serving Method:

Serve as an elegant appetizer or snack.

AIP COMPLIANT DESSERT RECIPES.

CAROB FUDGE.

Prep Time: 10 minutes

Cooking Time: 0 minutes

Ingredients:

- 1/2 cup coconut oil, melted
- 1/2 cup carob powder
- 1/4 cup honey or maple syrup
- 1/2 teaspoon vanilla extract (AIP-friendly)

Directions:

- Prepare a small baking dish with parchment paper.
- In a bowl, mix together melted coconut oil, carob powder, honey or maple syrup, and vanilla extract until smooth.
- Pour the mixture into the prepared baking dish and spread it evenly.
- Place in the refrigerator for at least 1 hour, or until set.
- Cut into squares and serve.

Serving Method:

Serve chilled.

COCONUT MACAROONS.

Prep Time: 10 minutes

Cooking Time: 20 minutes

Ingredients:

- 2 cups shredded coconut
- 1/4 cup coconut oil, melted
- 1/4 cup honey or maple syrup
- 1 teaspoon vanilla extract (AIP-friendly)

Directions:

- Preheat oven to 350°F (175°C) and set a baking sheet with parchment paper.
- In a bowl, mix together shredded coconut, melted coconut oil, honey or maple syrup, and vanilla extract until well combined.
- Use a cookie scoop to form the mixture into balls and place them on the prepared baking sheet.
- Bake for 15-20 minutes, or until golden brown.

Serving Method:

Serve at room temperature.

AIP BANANA BREAD.

Prep Time: 15 minutes

Cooking Time: 45 minutes

Ingredients:

- 2 ripe bananas, mashed
- 1/4 cup coconut oil, melted

- 1/4 cup coconut flour
- 1/4 cup tapioca flour
- 1/2 teaspoon baking soda
- 1/2 teaspoon cinnamon
- Pinch of salt

Directions:

- Preheat oven to 350°F (175°C) and oil a loaf pan.
- -In a bowl, mix together mashed bananas and melted coconut oil.
- Add coconut flour, tapioca flour, baking soda, cinnamon, and salt. Mix until well combined.
- Pour the batter into the oiled loaf pan.
- Bake for 40-45 minutes, or until a toothpick stuck into the center comes out clean.
- Allow to cool before slicing and serving.

Serving Method:

Serve at room temperature.

TIGER NUT FLOUR COOKIES.

Prep Time: 15 minutes

Cooking Time: 12 minutes

Ingredients:

- 1 cup tiger nut flour
- 1/4 cup coconut oil, melted
- 1/4 cup honey or maple syrup
- 1/2 teaspoon vanilla extract (AIP-friendly)

Directions:

- Preheat oven to 350°F (175°C) and set a baking sheet with parchment paper.
- In a bowl, mix together tiger nut flour, melted coconut oil, honey or maple syrup, and vanilla extract until well combined.
- Use a cookie scoop to form the mixture into balls and place them on the prepared baking sheet.
- Flatten each ball with a fork.
- Bake for 10-12 minutes, or until lightly golden.

Serving Method:

Serve at room temperature.

BAKED APPLES WITH CINNAMON.

Prep Time: 10 minutes

Cooking Time: 30 minutes

Ingredients:

- 4 apples, cored
- 2 tablespoons coconut oil, melted
- 2 tablespoons of honey or maple syrup
- 1 teaspoon cinnamon

Directions:

- Preheat oven to 350°F (175°C) and line a baking dish with parchment paper.
- Place cored apples in the baking dish.

- In a small bowl, mix together melted coconut oil, honey or maple syrup, and cinnamon.
- Spoon the mixture into the center of each apple.
- Bake for 25-30 minutes, or until apples are tender.

Serving Method:

Serve warm.

AIP PUMPKIN PIE.

Prep Time: 20 minutes

Cooking Time: 50 minutes

Ingredients:

- 1 can (15 ounces) of pumpkin puree
- 1/2 cup coconut milk
- 1/2 cup maple syrup
- 2 teaspoons pumpkin pie spice
- 1/2 teaspoon salt
- 2 tablespoons coconut flour
- 2 tablespoons gelatin
- 1/4 cup water

Directions:

- Preheat oven to 350°F (175°C).
- In a saucepan, combine pumpkin puree, coconut milk, maple syrup, pumpkin pie spice, and salt. Cook over low heat until it's heated through.

- In a small bowl, mix coconut flour with a small amount of water to form a paste. Add this to the pumpkin mixture and stir until thickened.
- In another small bowl, mix gelatin with water. Allow to sit for a few minutes to bloom. Add this to the pumpkin mixture and stir until well combined.
- Pour the pumpkin mixture into a prepared pie crust and smoothen the top.
- Bake for 50 minutes, or until set.

Serving Method:

Serve chilled.

COCONUT FLOUR CAKE.

Prep Time: 15 minutes

Cooking Time: 30 minutes

Ingredients:

- 1/2 cup coconut flour
- 1/4 cup tapioca flour
- 1/2 teaspoon baking soda
- Pinch of salt
- 4 eggs
- 1/2 cup coconut oil, melted
- 1/2 cup maple syrup
- 1 teaspoon vanilla extract (AIP-friendly)

Directions:

- Preheat oven to 350°F (175°C) and grease a cake pan.

- In a bowl, whisk coconut flour, tapioca flour, baking soda, and salt together.
- In another bowl, whisk together eggs, melted coconut oil, maple syrup, and vanilla extract.
- Gradually add the wet ingredients to the dry ingredients, thoroughly stir until well combined.
- Pour the batter into the prepared cake pan.
- Bake for 25-30 minutes, or until a toothpick put into the center comes out clean.

Serving Method:

Serve at room temperature.

MIXED BERRY SORBET.

Prep Time: 10 minutes

Cooking Time: 0 minutes

Ingredients:

- 2 cups of mixed berries (strawberries, blueberries, raspberries)
- 1/4 cup coconut milk
- 2 tablespoons of honey or maple syrup

Directions:

- In a blender, combine mixed berries, coconut milk, and honey or maple syrup.
- Blend until smooth.
- Pour the mixture into a shallow dish and freeze for 2-3 hours, stirring every 30 minutes to break up ice crystals.

Serving Method:

- Serve frozen.

AIP LEMON BARS.

Prep Time: 20 minutes

Cooking Time: 30 minutes

Ingredients:

For the crust:

- 1 cup coconut flour
- 1/2 cup coconut oil, melted
- 1/4 cup maple syrup
- Pinch of salt

For the filling:

- 1/2 cup lemon juice
- Zest of 1 lemon
- 1/2 cup honey or maple syrup
- 4 eggs
- 1/4 cup coconut flour

Directions:

- Preheat oven to 350°F (175°C) and grease a baking dish.
- In a bowl, combine coconut flour, melted coconut oil, maple syrup, and salt. Press the mixture into the bottom of the already greased baking dish.
- Bake the crust for 10-15 minutes, or until lightly golden.

- In another bowl, whisk together lemon juice, lemon zest, honey or maple syrup, eggs, and coconut flour.
- Pour the filling over the baked crust.
- Bake for 15-20 minutes, or until the filling is set.
- Let cool before slicing into bars.

Serving Method:

Serve chilled.

SWEET POTATO BROWNIES.

Prep Time: 20 minutes

Cooking Time: 30 minutes

Ingredients:

- 1 cup mashed sweet potato
- 1/2 cup coconut flour
- 1/2 cup cocoa powder
- 1/2 cup maple syrup
- 1/4 cup coconut oil, melted
- 2 teaspoons vanilla extract (AIP-friendly)
- 1/2 teaspoon baking soda
- Pinch of salt

Directions:

- Preheat oven to 350°F (175°C) and grease a baking dish.
- In a bowl, combine mashed sweet potato, coconut flour, cocoa powder, maple syrup, melted coconut oil, vanilla extract, baking soda, and salt. Mix until well combined.

- Pour the batter into the prepared baking dish and smooth the top.
- Bake for 25-30 minutes, or until a toothpick put into the center comes out clean.
- Let cool before serving.

Serving method:

Serve at room temperature.

TIGER NUT FLOUR PANCAKES.

Prep Time: 10 minutes

Cooking Time: 10 minutes

Ingredients:

- 1/2 cup tiger nut flour
- 1/4 cup coconut milk
- 2 eggs
- 1 tablespoon coconut oil, melted
- 1 tablespoon of honey (or maple syrup)
- 1/2 teaspoon baking soda
- Pinch of salt

Directions:

- In a bowl, whisk together tiger nut flour, coconut milk, eggs, melted coconut oil, honey or maple syrup, baking soda, and salt until smooth.
- Heat a skillet over medium heat and grease with coconut oil.
- Pour batter onto the skillet to form pancakes.

- Cook for 2-3 minutes per side, or until golden brown.

Serving Method:

Serve warm with your preferred or favorite toppings.

BLUEBERRY COCONUT POPSICLES.

Prep Time: 10 minutes

Freezing Time: 4 hours

Ingredients:

- 1 can (that is 13.5 ounces) of coconut milk
- 1 cup blueberries
- 2 tablespoons of honey or maple syrup

Directions:

- In a blender, combine coconut milk, blueberries, and honey or maple syrup.
- Blend until smooth.
- Pour into popsicles molds.
- Insert sticks and freeze for at least 4 hours, or until solid.
- Run warm water over the molds to release the popsicles.

Serving Method:

Serve frozen.

CINNAMON RAISIN COOKIES.

Prep Time: 15 minutes

Cooking Time: 15 minutes

Ingredients:

- 1 cup coconut flour
- 1/2 cup coconut oil, melted
- 1/2 cup honey or maple syrup
- 2 eggs
- 1 teaspoon cinnamon
- 1/2 cup raisins

Directions:

- Preheat oven to 350°F (175°C) and set a baking sheet with parchment paper.
- In a bowl, mix together coconut flour, melted coconut oil, honey or maple syrup, eggs, and cinnamon until well combined.
- Fold in raisins.
- Use a cookie scoop to form the mixture into balls and place them on the prepared baking sheet.
- Flatten each ball with a fork.
- Bake for 12-15 minutes, or until lightly golden.
- Let cool before serving.

Serving Method:

Serve at room temperature.

AIP APPLE CRISP.

Prep Time: 15 minutes

Cooking Time: 40 minutes

Ingredients:

For the filling:

- 4 apples, peeled and sliced
- 1/4 cup honey or maple syrup
- 1 tablespoon lemon juice
- 1 teaspoon cinnamon

For the topping:

- 1 cup shredded coconut
- 1/2 cup coconut flour
- 1/2 cup coconut oil, melted
- 1/4 cup honey or maple syrup
- 1 teaspoon cinnamon

Directions:

- Preheat oven to 350°F (175°C) and grease a baking dish.
- In a bowl, combine sliced apples, honey or maple syrup, lemon juice, and cinnamon. Mix until apples are coated.
- Spread the apple mixture in the prepared baking dish.
- In another bowl, mix together shredded coconut, coconut flour, melted coconut oil, honey or maple syrup, and cinnamon until crumbly.
- Sprinkle the topping over the apples.
- Bake for 35-40 minutes, or until the topping is golden brown and the apples are tender.
- Let cool slightly before serving.

Serving Method:

Serve warm.

COCONUT MILK PANNA COTTA.

Prep Time: 10 minutes

Cooking Time: 5 minutes

Chilling Time: 4 hours

Ingredients:

- 1 can (or 13.5 ounces) of coconut milk
- 1/4 cup honey or maple syrup
- 2 teaspoons gelatin
- 2 tablespoons water
- 1 teaspoon vanilla extract (AIP-friendly)

Directions:

- In a saucepan, heat coconut milk and honey or maple syrup over medium heat until warm.
- In a small bowl, add gelatin with water and stir. Allow to sit for a few minutes to bloom.
- Add the bloomed gelatin to the warm coconut milk mixture and stir until dissolved.
- Remove from heat and stir in vanilla extract.
- Pour the mixture into ramekins or molds.
- Refrigerate for at least 4 hours, or until set.

Serving Method:

Serve chilled, topped with fresh berries if desired.

PUMPKIN SPICE MUFFINS.

Prep Time: 15 minutes

Cooking Time: 25 minutes

Ingredients:

- 1/2 cup pumpkin puree
- 1/4 cup coconut oil, melted
- 1/4 cup maple syrup
- 2 eggs
- 1 teaspoon vanilla extract (AIP-friendly)
- 1/2 cup coconut flour
- 1/2 teaspoon baking soda
- 1 teaspoon cinnamon
- 1/2 teaspoon ginger
- 1/4 teaspoon nutmeg
- Pinch of cloves

Directions:

- Preheat oven to 350°F (175°C) and set a muffin tin with paper liners.
- In a bowl, mix together pumpkin puree, melted coconut oil, maple syrup, eggs, and vanilla extract until well combined.
- Add coconut flour, baking soda, cinnamon, ginger, nutmeg, and cloves. Mix until smooth.
- Evenly divide the batter evenly among the muffin cups.
- Bake for 20-25 minutes, or until a toothpick put into the center comes out clean.
- Let cool before serving.

Serving Method:

Serve at room temperature.

AIP CHOCOLATE CHIP COOKIES.

Prep Time: 15 minutes

Cooking Time: 10 minutes

Ingredients:

- 1/2 cup coconut flour
- 1/4 cup coconut oil, melted
- 1/4 cup maple syrup
- 1/2 teaspoon baking soda
- Pinch of salt
- 1/4 cup carob chips or AIP-friendly chocolate chips

Directions:

- Preheat oven to 350°F (175°C) and set a baking sheet with parchment paper.
- In a bowl, mix together coconut flour, melted coconut oil, maple syrup, baking soda, and salt until well combined.
- Fold in carob chips or chocolate chips.
- Use a cookie scoop to form the mixture into balls and place them on the prepared baking sheet.
- Flatten each ball with a fork.
- Bake for 8-10 minutes, or until lightly golden or browned.
- Let cool before serving.

Serving Method:

Serve at room temperature.

STRAWBERRY COCONUT ICE CREAM.

Preparation Time: 10 minutes

Freezing Time: 4 hours

Ingredients:

- 1 can of (13.5 ounces) coconut milk
- 2 cups frozen strawberries
- 1/4 cup honey or maple syrup

Directions:

- In a blender, combine coconut milk, frozen strawberries, and honey or maple syrup.
- Blend until smooth.
- Pour the mixture into a shallow dish and freeze for at least 4 hours, stirring every 30 minutes to break up ice crystals.

Serving Method:

Serve frozen.

LEMON COCONUT BLISS BALLS.

Prep Time: 15 minutes

Chilling Time: 30 minutes

Ingredients:

- 1 cup shredded coconut
- 1/4 cup coconut oil, melted
- 2 tablespoons of honey (or maple syrup)
- Zest of 1 lemon
- Juice of 1/2 lemon

Directions:

- In a food processor, combine shredded coconut, melted coconut oil, honey or maple syrup, lemon zest, and lemon juice. Pulse until well combined.
- Roll the mixture into balls and place them on a baking sheet lined with parchment paper.
- -Refrigerate for at least 30 minutes, or until firm.

Serving Method:

Serve chilled.

CAROB BARK.

Prep Time: 15 minutes

Chilling Time: 1 hour

Ingredients:

- 1/2 cup coconut oil, melted
- 1/2 cup carob powder
- 1/4 cup honey or maple syrup
- 1/4 cup shredded coconut

Directions:

- Set a baking sheet with parchment paper.
- In a bowl, mix together melted coconut oil, carob powder, honey or maple syrup, and shredded coconut until smooth.
- -Pour the mixture onto the prepared baking sheet and spread it evenly.
- Place in the refrigerator for at least 1 hour, or until set.

-   Break into pieces before serving.

Serving Method:

Serve chilled.

AIP FRIENDLY DRINK RECIPES.

GINGER TURMERIC TEA.

Prep Time: 5 minutes

Cooking Time: 10 minutes

Ingredients:

- 2 cups water
- 1-inch piece of ginger, peeled and sliced
- 1-inch piece of turmeric, peeled and chopped
- 1 tablespoon honey (optional)

Directions:

- Heat water in a small saucepan, until it boils.
- Add ginger and turmeric to the boiling water.
- Reduce the heat and allow to simmer for 10 minutes.
- Strain the tea and stir in honey if desired.

Serving Method:

Serve hot.

AIP GREEN SMOOTHIE (USING AIP-FRIENDLY INGREDIENTS)

Prep Time: 5 minutes

Cooking Time: 0 minutes

Ingredients:

- 1 cup coconut milk
- 1/2 avocado
- 1 handful spinach
- 1/2 cucumber, peeled and chopped
- 1 tablespoon fresh mint leaves
- 1 tablespoon honey (optional)

Directions:

- Pour all ingredients in a blender.
- Blend until smooth.

Serving Method:

Serve cold.

LEMON BALM TEA.

Prep Time: 5 minutes

Cooking Time: 5 minutes

Ingredients:

- 2 cups water
- 1/4 cup of fresh lemon balm leaves
- 1 tablespoon honey (optional)

Directions:

- Heat water in a small saucepan, and let it boil.
- Add lemon balm leaves to the boiling water.
- Remove from heat and let steep for 5 minutes.
- Strain the tea and stir in honey if desired.

Serving Method:

Serve hot or cold.

COCONUT MILK CHAI LATTE (USING AIP-APPROVED SPICES).

Prep Time: 5 minutes

Cooking Time: 5 minutes

Ingredients:

- 1 cup coconut milk
- 1/2 teaspoon ground cinnamon
- 1/4 teaspoon ground ginger
- 1/4 teaspoon ground cloves
- 1/4 teaspoon ground cardamom
- 1/4 teaspoon vanilla extract (AIP-friendly)
- 1 tablespoon honey (optional)

Directions:

- In a small saucepan, combine coconut milk, cinnamon, ginger, cloves, and cardamom.
- Bring to a simmer low medium heat.
- Remove from heat and stir in vanilla extract and honey if desired.

Serving Method:

Serve hot.

WATERMELON MINT COOLER.

Prep Time: 10 minutes

Cooking Time: 0 minutes

Ingredients:

- 4 cups cubed watermelon
- 1/4 cup fresh mint leaves
- 1 tablespoon lime juice
- Ice cubes

Directions:

- In a blender, combine watermelon, mint leaves, and lime juice.
- Blend until smooth.
- Strain the mixture to get rid of any pulp.
- Serve over ice.

Serving Method:

Serve cold.

HERBAL INFUSION (E.G., CHAMOMILE, PEPPERMINT).

Prep Time: 5 minutes

Cooking Time: 5 minutes

Ingredients:

- 2 cups water
- 2 tablespoons dried chamomile flowers or peppermint leaves

Directions:

- Heat water in small saucepan until it boils.
- Add chamomile flowers or peppermint leaves to the boiling water.
- Remove from heat and let steep for 5 minutes.
- Strain the infusion.

Serving Method:

Serve hot or cold.

AIP GOLDEN MILK (USING COCONUT MILK AND TURMERIC).

Prep Time: 5 minutes

Cooking Time: 5 minutes

Ingredients:

- 1 cup coconut milk
- 1/2 teaspoon ground turmeric
- 1/4 teaspoon ground ginger
- Pinch of ground cinnamon
- Pinch of ground cloves
- Pinch of ground black pepper
- 1 tablespoon honey (optional)

Directions:

- In a small saucepan, add coconut milk, turmeric, ginger, cinnamon, cloves, and black pepper.
- Bring to a simmer over low heat.
- Remove from heat and stir in honey if desired.

Serving Method:

Serve hot.

CUCUMBER MINT INFUSED WATER.

Prep Time: 5 minutes

Cooking Time: 0 minutes

Ingredients:

- 4 cups water
- 1 cucumber, sliced
- 1/4 cup fresh mint leaves

Directions:

- In a pitcher, combine water, cucumber slices, and mint leaves.
- Refrigerate for at least 1 hour to allow flavors to infuse.

Serving Method:

Serve cold.

BLUEBERRY GINGER SMOOTHIE.

Prep Time: 5 minutes

Cooking Time: 0 minutes

Ingredients:

- 1 cup coconut milk

- 1/2 cup blueberries
- 1/2 banana
- 1 tablespoon fresh ginger, grated
- 1 tablespoon honey (optional)

Directions:

- Pour all ingredients in a blender.
- Blend until smooth.

Serving Method:

Serve cold.

HIBISCUS ROSEHIP TEA.

Prep Time: 5 minutes

Cooking Time: 10 minutes

Ingredients:

- 2 cups water
- 2 tablespoons dried hibiscus flowers
- 1 tablespoon dried rosehips

Directions:

- Heat water in a small saucepan until it boils.
- Add hibiscus flowers and rosehips to the boiling water.
- Remove from heat and let steep for 5-10 minutes.
- Strain the tea.

Serving Method:

Serve hot or cold.

AIP HOT COCOA (USING CAROB POWDER AND COCONUT MILK).

Prep Time: 5 minutes

Cooking Time: 5 minutes

Ingredients:

- 1 cup coconut milk
- 1 tablespoon carob powder
- 1 tablespoon honey (optional)

Directions:

- In a small saucepan, heat coconut milk over medium heat.
- Whisk in carob powder until smooth.
- Add honey if desired and stir until dissolved.

Serving Method:

Serve hot.

MANGO PINEAPPLE SMOOTHIE.

Prep Time: 5 minutes

Cooking Time: 0 minutes

Ingredients:

- 1 cup coconut milk
- 1/2 cup mango chunks

- 1/2 cup pineapple chunks

Directions:

- Pour all the ingredients in a blender.
- Blend until smooth.

Serving Method:

Serve cold.

DANDELION ROOT TEA.

Prep Time: 5 minutes

Cooking Time: 10 minutes

Ingredients:

- 2 cups water
- 2 tablespoons dried dandelion root

Directions:

- Heat water in a small saucepan until it boils.
- Add dried dandelion root to the boiling water.
- Reduce heat and simmer for 5-10 minutes.
- Strain the tea.

Serving Method:

Serve hot or cold.

COCONUT WATER ELECTROLYTE DRINK.

Prep Time: 5 minutes

Cooking Time: 0 minutes

Ingredients:

- 1 cup coconut water
- 1/4 teaspoon sea salt
- 1/4 teaspoon honey (optional)

Directions:

- In a glass, combine coconut water, sea salt, and honey.
- Stir until salt and honey are dissolved.

Serving Method:

Serve cold.

AIP STRAWBERRY BANANA SMOOTHIE.

Prep Time: 5 minutes

Cooking Time: 0 minutes

Ingredients:

- 1 cup coconut milk
- 1/2 cup strawberries
- 1/2 banana

Directions:

- Pour all ingredients in a blender.
- Blend until smooth.

Serving Method:

Serve cold.

LAVENDER LEMONADE.

Prep Time: 10 minutes

Cooking Time: 0 minutes

Ingredients:

- 1/2 cup fresh lemon juice
- 4 cups water
- 1/4 cup honey (or to taste)
- 1 tablespoon dried lavender flowers

Directions:

- In a small saucepan, combine 1 cup of water and dried lavender flowers. Bring to a simmer and let it simmer for 5 minutes. Remove from heat and let it cool.
- In a pitcher, combine lemon juice, honey, lavender-infused water, and the remaining 3 cups of water. Stir until the honey is dissolved.
- Refrigerate until cold.

Serving Method:

Serve over ice, garnished with a slice of lemon and a sprig of fresh lavender.

AIP ICED HERBAL CHAI.

Prep Time: 5 minutes

Cooking Time: 10 minutes

Ingredients:

- 4 cups water
- 1 tablespoon AIP-friendly chai spices (such as cinnamon, ginger, cloves, cardamom)
- 1 tablespoon honey (optional)

Directions:

- Heat water in a small saucepan until it boils.
- Add chai spices to the boiling water.
- Reduce heat and simmer for 5-10 minutes.
- Remove from heat and let it cool.
- Strain the chai mixture and discard the spices.
- Sweeten with honey if desired.
- Refrigerate until cold.

Serving Method:

Serve over ice.

BERRY HIBISCUS ICED TEA.

Prep Time: 10 minutes

Cooking Time: 0 minutes

Ingredients:

- 4 cups water
- 2 hibiscus tea bags
- 1 cup of mixed berries (like strawberries, blueberries, raspberries)
- 1 tablespoon honey (optional)

Directions:

- In a large pitcher, steep hibiscus tea bags in hot water for 5-10 minutes.
- Remove the tea bags and let the tea cool.
- In a blender, blend mixed berries until smooth.
- Add blended berries to the cooled tea and mix well.
- Sweeten with honey if desired.
- Refrigerate until cold.

Serving Method:

Serve over ice.

AIP PUMPKIN SPICE LATTE (USING COCONUT MILK AND AIP SPICES).

Prep Time: 10 minutes

Cooking Time: 5 minutes

Ingredients:

- 1 cup coconut milk
- 1/4 cup pumpkin puree
- 1 tablespoon of honey (or to taste)
- 1/2 teaspoon ground cinnamon
- 1/4 teaspoon ground ginger
- Pinch of ground cloves
- Pinch of ground nutmeg

Directions:

- In a small saucepan, combine coconut milk, pumpkin puree, honey, and spices.

- Heat over medium heat, whisking constantly, until heated through.
- Remove from heat and froth with a frother if desired.

Serving Method:

Serve hot, topped with a sprinkle of cinnamon.

SPARKLING WATER WITH FRESH LEMON OR LIME JUICE.

Prep Time: 5 minutes

Cooking Time: 0 minutes

Ingredients:

- Sparkling water
- Fresh lemon or lime juice

Directions:

- Fill a glass with ice.
- Pour sparkling water over the ice.
- Squeeze fresh lemon or lime juice into the water.
- Stir gently.

Serving Method:

Serve cold.

VEGETARIAN AND VEGAN AIP RECIPES.

ROASTED VEGETABLE SALAD.

Prep Time: 15 minutes

Cooking Time: 30 minutes

Ingredients:

- Assorted vegetables (such as bell peppers, zucchini, and carrots), chopped
- 2 tablespoons olive oil
- Salt and pepper to taste
- Mixed greens
- AIP-friendly salad dressing

Directions:

- Preheat oven to 400°F (200°C).
- Toss chopped vegetables with olive oil, salt, and pepper.
- Spread vegetables on a baking sheet and roast for 25-30 minutes, or until tender and lightly browned.
- Serve roasted vegetables over mixed greens and drizzle with AIP-friendly salad dressing.

Serving method:

Serve hot or cold as a salad.

CAULIFLOWER RICE STIR-FRY.

Prep Time: 10 minutes

Cooking Time: 15 minutes

Ingredients:

- 1 head cauliflower, riced
- 2 tablespoons coconut oil
- 1 onion, chopped
- 2 garlic cloves, minced
- Assorted vegetables (such as bell peppers, broccoli, and mushrooms), chopped
- 2 tablespoons coconut aminos
- Salt and pepper to taste

Directions:

- In a large skillet, heat coconut oil over medium heat.
- Add onion and garlic then cook until onion is soft.
- Add assorted vegetables to the skillet. Cook until vegetables are tender.
- Stir in cauliflower rice and coconut aminos. Cook for an additional 5 minutes.

Serving Method:

Serve hot as a main dish or side.

ZUCCHINI NOODLES WITH PESTO.

Prep Time: 15 minutes

Cooking Time: 0 minutes

Ingredients:

- 2-3 zucchinis, spiralized into noodles
- AIP-friendly pesto sauce

Directions:

- Spiralize zucchinis into noodles.
- Toss zucchini noodles with AIP-friendly pesto sauce.

Serving Method:

Serve cold as a refreshing pasta alternative.

SWEET POTATO AND APPLE SOUP.

Prep Time: 15 minutes

Cooking Time: 30 minutes

Ingredients:

- 2 sweet potatoes, peeled and diced
- 2 apples, peeled, cored, and well chopped
- 1 onion, chopped
- 2 garlic cloves, minced
- 4 cups vegetable broth
- 1 teaspoon cinnamon
- Salt and pepper to taste

Directions:

- In a large pot, combine sweet potatoes, apples, onion, garlic, vegetable broth, cinnamon, salt, and pepper.
- Bring to a boil, then reduce heat and simmer for 20-25 minutes, or until sweet potatoes are tender.

- To make the soup smooth, make use of an immersion blender to blend it.

Serving Method:

Serve hot, garnished with a sprinkle of cinnamon.

COCONUT CURRY VEGETABLES.

Prep Time: 15 minutes

Cooking Time: 20 minutes

Ingredients:

- Assorted vegetables (such as cauliflower, bell peppers, and snap peas), chopped
- 1 can coconut milk
- 2 tablespoons curry powder (AIP-friendly)
- Salt and pepper to taste

Directions:

- In a large skillet, combine vegetables, coconut milk, curry powder, salt, and pepper.
- Bring to a simmer and cook for 15-20 minutes, or until vegetables are tender.

Serving Method:

Serve hot over cauliflower rice or with AIP-friendly naan bread.

PLANTAIN PIZZA WITH AIP-FRIENDLY TOPPINGS.

Prep Time: 15 minutes

Cooking Time: 25 minutes

Ingredients:

- 2 ripe plantains
- 2 tablespoons coconut oil
- AIP-friendly pizza sauce
- AIP-friendly toppings (such as cooked chicken, vegetables, and herbs)

Directions:

- Preheat oven to 375°F (190°C).
- Peel the plantains and slice them lengthwise.
- Heat coconut oil in a skillet over low heat.
- Fry plantain slices until golden brown, about 2-3 minutes per side.
- Place fried plantain slices on a baking sheet.
- Top plantain slices with pizza sauce and AIP-friendly toppings.
- Bake in the preheated oven for 15-20 minutes, or until toppings are heated through.

Serving Method:

Serve hot, sliced into pieces.

STUFFED BELL PEPPERS WITH AIP-COMPLIANT FILLING.

Prep Time: 20 minutes

Cooking Time: 30 minutes

Ingredients:

- 4 bell peppers, cut into half and seeded
- 1 pound ground meat (such as turkey or beef)
- 1 onion, chopped
- 2 garlic cloves, minced
- 1 cup chopped vegetables (such as carrots, zucchini, and mushrooms)
- 1 can diced tomatoes
- 1 teaspoon dried herbs (such as oregano and basil)
- Salt and pepper to taste

Directions:

- Preheat oven to 375°F (190°C).
- In a skillet, cook ground meat over medium heat until browned.
- In the skillet, add onion and garlic and cook until the onion is soft.
- Stir in chopped vegetables, diced tomatoes, dried herbs, salt, and pepper. Cook for an additional 5 minutes.
- Fill each bell pepper half with the meat mixture.
- Put the stuffed bell peppers into a baking dish.
- Bake in the preheated oven for 25-30 minutes, or until peppers are tender.

Serving Method:

- Serve hot, with a side salad.

MUSHROOM AND SPINACH STIR-FRY.

Preparation Time: 10 minutes

Cooking Time: 10 minutes

Ingredients:

- - **Directions:** 2 tablespoons coconut oil
- 8 ounces mushrooms, sliced
- 2 garlic cloves, minced
- 4 cups spinach
- 2 tablespoons coconut aminos
- Salt and pepper to taste

Directions:

- In a large skillet, heat coconut oil over medium heat.
- Add mushrooms to the skillet. Cook until mushrooms are tender.
- Stir in garlic and allow to cook for an additional minute.
- Add spinach and coconut aminos to the skillet. Cook until spinach is wilted.
- Season with salt and pepper.

Serving Method:

Serve as a hot side dish or over cauliflower rice.

LENTIL-FREE VEGETABLE SOUP.

Prep Time: 15 minutes

Cooking Time: 30 minutes

Ingredients:

- 2 tablespoons olive oil
- 1 onion, chopped
- 2 carrots, chopped
- 2 celery stalks, chopped
- 2 garlic cloves, minced
- 6 cups vegetable broth
- 1 can diced tomatoes
- 2 cups chopped vegetables (such as zucchini, bell peppers, and green beans)
- 1 teaspoon dried herbs (such as thyme and rosemary)
- Salt and pepper to taste

Directions:

- Heat up olive oil in a large pot over low heat.
- Add onion, carrots, celery, and garlic to the pot. Cook until vegetables are tender.
- Stir in vegetable broth, diced tomatoes, chopped vegetables, dried herbs, salt, and pepper.
- Bring to a boil, then reduce heat and simmer for 20-25 minutes, or until vegetables are tender.

Serving Method:

Serve hot and garnish with fresh herbs if preferred.

PORTOBELLO MUSHROOM BURGERS WITH AIP-FRIENDLY CONDIMENTS.

Prep Time: 15 minutes

Cooking Time: 15 minutes

Ingredients:

- 4 large portobello mushrooms
- 2 tablespoons olive oil
- AIP-friendly burger toppings (such as lettuce, tomato, avocado, and AIP-friendly mayo)

Directions:

- Preheat grill or grill pan over low heat.
- Brush portobello mushrooms with olive oil.
- Grill mushrooms for 4-5 minutes per side, or until tender.
- Assemble burgers with grilled portobello mushrooms and AIP-friendly condiments.

Serving Method:

Serve hot, with any remaining toppings on the side.

VEGGIE STIR-FRY WITH COCONUT AMINOS.

Prep Time: 15 minutes

Cooking Time: 10 minutes

Ingredients:

- 2 tablespoons coconut oil
- 1 onion, sliced
- 2 bell peppers, sliced
- 2 cups broccoli florets
- 1 cup snap peas
- 1/4 cup coconut aminos
- Salt and pepper to taste

Directions:

- In a large skillet, heat coconut oil over medium heat.
- Add onion to the skillet. Cook until onion is soft.
- Add bell peppers, broccoli, and snap peas to the skillet. Cook until vegetables are tender-crisp.
- Stir in coconut aminos, salt, and pepper. Cook for an additional 2-3 minutes.

Serving Method:

Serve hot as a side dish or with cauliflower rice.

COCONUT MILK-BASED VEGETABLE CURRY.

Prep Time: 20 minutes

Cooking Time: 25 minutes

Ingredients:

- 2 tablespoons coconut oil
- 1 onion, chopped
- 2 garlic cloves, minced
- 1 tablespoon ginger, minced
- 2 tablespoons curry powder (AIP-friendly)
- 1 can coconut milk
- 4 cups chopped vegetables (such as carrots, potatoes, and peas)
- Salt and pepper to taste

Directions:

- Heat up coconut oil over low heat in a large pot.

- Add onion, garlic, and ginger to the pot. Cook until onion is soft.
- Stir in curry powder and cook for an additional minute.
- Add coconut milk and chopped vegetables to the pot. Bring to a simmer and cook for 15-20 minutes, or until vegetables are tender.
- Season with salt and pepper.

Serving Method:

Serve hot, over cauliflower rice or with AIP-friendly naan bread.

AIP RATATOUILLE.

Prep Time: 20 minutes

Cooking Time: 40 minutes

Ingredients:

- 2 tablespoons olive oil
- 1 onion, chopped
- 2 garlic cloves, minced
- 1 eggplant, diced
- 2 zucchinis, diced
- 1 bell pepper, diced
- 1 can diced tomatoes
- 1 teaspoon dried herbs (like basil and thyme)
- Salt and pepper to taste

Directions:

- Heat up olive oil over low heat in a large pot.

- Add onion and garlic to the pot. Cook until onion is soft.

- Add eggplant, zucchinis, and bell pepper to the pot. Cook for 10 minutes, stirring occasionally.
- Stir in diced tomatoes, dried herbs, salt, and pepper. Cook for an additional 20-30 minutes, or until vegetables are tender.

Serving Method:

Serve hot and garnish with fresh herbs if preferred.

BEET AND APPLE SALAD.

Prep Time: 15 minutes

Cooking Time: 0 minutes

Ingredients:

- 2 beets, peeled and grated
- 1 apple, grated
- 1/4 cup chopped walnuts
- 2 tablespoons olive oil
- 1 tablespoon apple cider vinegar
- Salt and pepper to taste

Directions:

- In a bowl, combine grated beets, grated apple, and chopped walnuts.
- In a separate bowl, whisk together olive oil, apple cider vinegar, salt, and pepper.
- Pour dressing over the beet and apple mixture. Toss to combine.

Serving Method:

Serve cold as a refreshing side salad.

COCONUT-CAULIFLOWER MASH.

Prep Time: 10 minutes

Cooking Time: 15 minutes

Ingredients:

-   1 head cauliflower, chopped
-   1/2 cup coconut milk
-   2 tablespoons coconut oil
-   Salt and pepper to taste

Directions:

-   Steam cauliflower until tender.
-   In a food processor, combine steamed cauliflower, coconut milk, coconut oil, salt, and pepper. Blend until smooth.

Serving Method:

Serve hot as a creamy side dish.

AIP VEGGIE CHILI.

Prep Time: 20 minutes

Cooking Time: 30 minutes

Ingredients:

-   2 tablespoons coconut oil

- 1 onion, chopped
- 2 garlic cloves, minced
- 2 carrots, chopped
- 2 celery stalks, chopped
- 1 bell pepper, chopped
- 1 zucchini, chopped
- 1 can diced tomatoes
- 2 cups vegetable broth
- 1 tablespoon chili powder (AIP-friendly)
- 1 teaspoon dried herbs (such as oregano and basil)
- Salt and pepper to taste

Directions:

- Heat up coconut oil over low heat in a large pot.
- Add onion and garlic to the pot. Cook until onion is soft.
- Stir in carrots, celery, bell pepper, and zucchini. Cook for 5-7 minutes, or until vegetables are tender.
- Add diced tomatoes, vegetable broth, chili powder, dried herbs, salt, and pepper to the pot. Bring to a simmer then cook for about 15-20 minutes.

Serving Method:

Serve hot, garnished with chopped cilantro if desired.

SPAGHETTI SQUASH WITH AIP MARINARA SAUCE.

Prep Time: 10 minutes

Cooking Time: 40 minutes

Ingredients:

- 1 spaghetti squash, halved and seeded
- 2 tablespoons olive oil
- AIP-friendly marinara sauce

Directions:

- Preheat oven to 400°F (200°C).
- Place spaghetti squash halves on a baking sheet, cut side up. Sprinkle with olive oil, then season with salt and pepper.
- Roast spaghetti squash in the preheated oven for 30-40 minutes, or until tender.
- Use a fork to scrape the spaghetti squash flesh into strands.
- Serve spaghetti squash with AIP-friendly marinara sauce.

Serving Method:

Serve hot as a pasta alternative.

SWEET POTATO AND KALE HASH.

Prep Time: 15 minutes

Cooking Time: 20 minutes

Ingredients:

- 2 sweet potatoes, peeled and diced
- 2 tablespoons coconut oil
- 1 onion, chopped
- 2 garlic cloves, minced
- 4 cups chopped kale
- Salt and pepper to taste

Directions:

- In a large skillet, heat coconut oil over medium heat.
- Add sweet potatoes to the skillet. Cook until potatoes are soft and lightly browned for about 10-15 minutes.
- Add onion and garlic to the skillet and cook until the onion is soft.
- Stir in chopped kale and cook until kale is wilted.
- Season with salt and pepper.

Serving Method:

Serve hot as a side dish or topped with a fried egg for breakfast.

AIP VEGGIE SUSHI ROLLS WITH COCONUT AMINOS.

Prep Time: 30 minutes

Cooking Time: 0 minutes

Ingredients:

- Nori sheets
- 2 cups cauliflower rice
- Assorted vegetables (such as cucumber, avocado, and carrot), julienned
- Coconut aminos

Directions:

- Set a nori sheet on a bamboo sushi mat.
- Spread a thin layer of cauliflower rice over the nori sheet.
- Arrange julienned vegetables in a line across the cauliflower rice.

- Roll the nori sheet tightly using the bamboo mat.
- Slice the sushi roll into bite-sized pieces.

Serving Method:

Serve with coconut aminos for dipping.

ROASTED BRUSSELS SPROUTS WITH BALSAMIC GLAZE.

Prep Time: 10 minutes

Cooking Time: 30 minutes

Ingredients:

- 1 pound Brussels sprouts, trimmed and halved
- 2 tablespoons olive oil
- Salt and pepper to taste
- Balsamic glaze (AIP-friendly)

Directions:

- Preheat oven to 400°F (200°C).
- Toss Brussels sprouts with olive oil, salt, and pepper.
- Spread Brussels sprouts on a baking sheet in a single layer.
- Roast in the preheated oven for 25-30 minutes, or until Brussels sprouts are tender and lightly browned.
- Sprinkle with balsamic glaze before serving.

Serving Method:

Serve hot as a side dish.

POULTRY, MEAT AND POTATOES AIP RECIPES.

HERB ROASTED CHICKEN WITH SWEET POTATOES.

Prep Time: 15 minutes

Cooking Time: 1 hour

Ingredients:

- 4 chicken thighs
- 2 sweet potatoes, peeled and diced
- 2 tablespoons olive oil
- 1 teaspoon dried thyme
- 1 teaspoon dried rosemary
- 1 teaspoon dried sage
- Salt and pepper to taste

Directions:

- Preheat oven to 400°F (200°C).
- In a bowl, combine olive oil, thyme, rosemary, sage, salt, and pepper.
- Rub the chicken thighs and sweet potatoes with the herb mixture.
- Place chicken thighs and sweet potatoes on a baking sheet.
- Roast in the preheated oven for 45-60 minutes, or until chicken is cooked through and sweet potatoes are tender.

Serving Method:

Serve hot, with additional herbs for garnish if preferred.

AIP BEEF STEW.

Prep Time: 20 minutes

Cooking Time: 2 hours

Ingredients:

- 1 pound stewing beef, cubed
- 2 tablespoons coconut oil
- 3 carrots, chopped
- 3 celery stalks, chopped
- 1 onion, chopped
- 2 garlic cloves, minced
- 4 cups beef broth
- 1 teaspoon dried thyme
- 1 teaspoon dried rosemary
- Salt and pepper to taste

Directions:

- Heat up coconut oil over medium-high heat in a large pot.
- Add beef cubes and brown on all sides.
- Add carrots, celery, onion, and garlic to the pot.
- Pour in beef broth and add thyme, rosemary, salt, and pepper.
- Bring to a boil, then reduce heat and simmer for 1.5-2 hours, or until beef is tender.

Serving Method:

Serve hot and garnish with fresh herbs if preferred.

BAKED TURKEY MEATBALLS WITH AIP-FRIENDLY SAUCE.

Prep Time: 15 minutes

Cooking Time: 25 minutes

Ingredients:

- 1 pound ground turkey
- 1/2 onion, grated
- 1 garlic clove, minced
- 1/4 cup chopped fresh parsley
- 1/4 cup coconut flour
- Salt and pepper to taste
- AIP-friendly tomato sauce for serving

Directions:

- Preheat oven to 400°F (200°C) and line a baking sheet with parchment paper.
- In a bowl, combine ground turkey, grated onion, garlic, parsley, coconut flour, salt, and pepper. Mix well.
- Form the mixture into meatballs and place them on the prepared baking sheet.
- Bake in the preheated oven for 20-25 minutes, or until cooked through.

Serving Method:

Serve hot, with AIP-friendly tomato sauce for dipping or drizzling.

ROSEMARY GARLIC ROAST LAMB WITH ROASTED VEGETABLES.

Prep Time: 15 minutes

Cooking Time: 1 hour 30 minutes

Ingredients:

- 1 leg of lamb
- 4 garlic cloves, minced
- 2 tablespoons chopped fresh rosemary
- 2 tablespoons olive oil
- Salt and pepper to taste
- Assorted vegetables (carrots, potatoes, onions) for roasting

Directions:

- Preheat oven to 375°F (190°C).
- In a bowl, combine minced garlic, chopped rosemary, olive oil, salt, and pepper.
- Rub the mixture all over the leg of lamb.
- Place the lamb in a roasting pan and roast in the preheated oven for 1 hour 30 minutes, or until cooked to your desired doneness.
- In the last 30 minutes of cooking, add the assorted vegetables to the roasting pan and toss with the pan juices.

Serving Method:

Serve hot, with roasted vegetables on the side.

AIP Pork Tenderloin with Apple Compote.

Prep Time: 10 minutes

Cooking Time: 25 minutes

Ingredients:

- 1 pork tenderloin
- 2 tablespoons coconut oil
- 2 apples, peeled, cored, and sliced
- 1/2 teaspoon cinnamon
- 1/4 teaspoon nutmeg (omit for AIP)
- 1/4 cup apple juice

Directions:

- Preheat oven to 400°F (200°C).
- Season pork tenderloin with salt and pepper.
- In a skillet, heat coconut oil over medium-high heat.
- Sear the pork tenderloin on all sides until browned.
- Transfer the pork tenderloin to a baking dish and roast in the preheated oven for 20-25 minutes, or until cooked through.
- -While the pork is roasting, prepare the apple compote. In the same skillet used for searing the pork, add sliced apples, cinnamon, and apple juice. Cook over medium heat until apples are soft and the liquid has reduced, about 10 minutes.
- Serve the roasted pork tenderloin with the apple compote on top.

Serving Method:

Serve hot, with the apple compote spooned over the pork tenderloin.

BEEF AND SWEET POTATO SHEPHERD'S PIE.

Prep Time: 30 minutes

Cooking Time: 45 minutes

Ingredients:

- 1 pound ground beef
- 1 onion, chopped
- 2 carrots, chopped
- 2 celery stalks, chopped
- 2 garlic cloves, minced
- 1 cup beef broth
- 2 tablespoons tomato paste
- 2 teaspoons dried thyme
- Salt and pepper to taste
- 4 cups mashed sweet potatoes

Directions:

- Preheat oven to 400°F (200°C).
- In a skillet, cook ground beef over medium heat until browned.
- Add onion, carrots, celery, and garlic to the skillet. Cook until vegetables are tender.
- Stir in beef broth, tomato paste, thyme, salt, and pepper. Simmer for 5 minutes.
- Transfer beef mixture to a baking dish and top with mashed sweet potatoes.
- Bake in the preheated oven for 20-25 minutes, or until heated through and golden on top.

Serving Method:

Serve hot, scooping out portions with a spatula.

AIP CHICKEN CURRY WITH CAULIFLOWER RICE.

Prep Time: 15 minutes

Cooking Time: 30 minutes

Ingredients:

- 1 pound chicken breast, cubed
- 1 onion, chopped
- 2 garlic cloves, minced
- 1 tablespoon ginger, minced
- 1 tablespoon turmeric
- 1 tablespoon curry powder (AIP-friendly)
- 1 can coconut milk
- 1 cauliflower, riced

Directions:

- In a skillet, cook chicken over medium heat until browned.
- Add onion, garlic, ginger, turmeric, and curry powder to the skillet. Cook until onion is soft.
- Stir in coconut milk and simmer for 15 minutes.
- Meanwhile, steam cauliflower rice until tender.
- Serve chicken curry over cauliflower rice.

Serving Method:

With a side of cauliflower rice, serve hot.

LEMON HERB GRILLED CHICKEN WITH ROASTED CARROTS.

Prep Time: 15 minutes

Cooking Time: 25 minutes

Ingredients:

- 1 pound chicken breast
- 2 tablespoons olive oil
- 1 lemon, juiced
- 2 garlic cloves, minced
- 1 tablespoon of sliced fresh herbs (like rosemary, thyme, or parsley)
- Salt and pepper to taste
- 4 cups baby carrots

Directions:

- In a bowl, combine olive oil, lemon juice, garlic, herbs, salt, and pepper.
- Allow chicken to marinate in the mixture for at least 30 minutes.
- Preheat grill to medium-high heat.
- Grill chicken for 6-7 minutes per side, or until cooked through.
- Meanwhile, toss baby carrots with olive oil, salt, and pepper. Roast in the oven at 400°F (200°C) for 20 minutes.

Serving Method:

Serve hot, with a side of roasted carrots.

AIP MEATLOAF WITH MASHED SWEET POTATOES.

Prep Time: 15 minutes

Cooking Time: 1 hour

Ingredients:

- 1 pound ground beef
- 1 onion, chopped
- 2 garlic cloves, minced
- 1/2 cup coconut flour
- 1/4 cup coconut milk
- 2 tablespoons tomato paste
- 1 tablespoon dried thyme
- Salt and pepper to taste
- 4 cups mashed sweet potatoes

Directions:

- Preheat oven to 350°F (175°C).
- In a bowl, combine ground beef, onion, garlic, coconut flour, coconut milk, tomato paste, thyme, salt, and pepper.
- Form the mixture into a loaf and place in a baking dish.
- Bake in the preheated oven for 45-60 minutes, or until cooked through.

Serving Method:

Serve hot, slicing the meatloaf and serving with a scoop of mashed sweet potatoes.

GARLIC HERB ROASTED TURKEY BREAST WITH STEAMED BROCCOLI.

Prep Time: 15 minutes

Cooking Time: 1 hour 30 minutes

Ingredients:

- 1 turkey breast
- 2 tablespoons olive oil
- 3 garlic cloves, minced
- 1 tablespoon chopped fresh herbs (such as rosemary, thyme, or sage)
- Salt and pepper to taste
- 4 cups broccoli florets

Directions:

- Preheat oven to 325°F (165°C).
- In a bowl, combine olive oil, garlic, herbs, salt, and pepper.
- Rub the mixture in the bowl all over the turkey breast.
- Place the turkey breast in a roasting pan and roast in the preheated oven for 1 hour 30 minutes, or until cooked through.
- Steam broccoli until tender.

Serving Method:

Serve hot, slicing the turkey breast and serving with steamed broccoli.

BEEF AND CABBAGE STIR-FRY.

Prep Time: 15 minutes

Cooking Time: 15 minutes

Ingredients:

- 1 pound ground beef
- 1 onion, chopped
- 1 small cabbage, shredded
- 2 carrots, julienned
- 2 tablespoons coconut aminos
- 1 tablespoon apple cider vinegar
- 1 teaspoon ginger powder
- Salt and pepper to taste

Directions:

- Cook ground beef over low heat until browned in a skillet.
- Add onion, cabbage, and carrots to the skillet. Cook until vegetables are tender.
- Stir in coconut aminos, apple cider vinegar, ginger powder, salt, and pepper. Cook for an additional 5 minutes.

Serving Method:

Serve hot, on its own or over cauliflower rice.

AIP PULLED PORK WITH AIP BBQ SAUCE.

Prep Time: 10 minutes

Cooking Time: 8 hours

Ingredients:

- 2 pounds pork shoulder
- 1 onion, chopped
- 2 garlic cloves, minced
- 1 cup AIP BBQ sauce

Directions:

- Put pork shoulder in a slow cooker.
- Add onion and garlic to the slow cooker.
- Pour AIP BBQ sauce over the pork.
- Cook on low for 8 hours, or until pork is tender and easily shredded.

Serving Method:

Serve hot, shredded and mixed with the cooking juices and onions.

Note: The time it takes to prepare pulled pork with BBQ sauce can vary depending on the cooking method. Typically, it takes around 8 to 10 hours to cook pulled pork in a slow cooker or crockpot on low heat. However, if you're using a pressure cooker or Instant Pot, it can be done in about 2 to 3 hours. Keep in mind that marinating the pork beforehand and allowing time for it to rest after cooking can add extra time to the process.

ROASTED ASPARAGUS AND BAKED LEMON GARLIC SALMON.

Prep Time: 10 minutes

Cooking Time: 15 minutes

Ingredients:

- 4 salmon fillets
- 2 tablespoons olive oil
- 2 garlic cloves, minced
- 1 lemon, juiced and zested
- Salt and pepper to taste
- 1 pound asparagus, trimmed

Directions:

- Preheat oven to 400°F (200°C).
- Place salmon fillets on a baking sheet prepared with parchment paper.
- In a bowl, combine olive oil, garlic, lemon juice, lemon zest, salt, and pepper.
- Brush the mixture over the salmon fillets.
- Arrange asparagus on the baking sheet around the salmon.
- Bake in the preheated oven for 12-15 minutes, or until salmon is cooked through and asparagus is tender.

Serving Method:

Serve hot, garnished with freshly squeezed lemon juice.

AIP CHICKEN AND SWEET POTATO HASH.

Prep Time: 15 minutes

Cooking Time: 25 minutes

Ingredients:

- 1 pound chicken breast, cubed

- 2 sweet potatoes, peeled and
- 1 onion, chopped
- 2 garlic cloves, minced
- 1 teaspoon dried thyme
- Salt and pepper to taste

Directions:

- Cook chicken over low heat until browned in a skillet.
- Add sweet potatoes, onion, garlic, thyme, salt, and pepper to the skillet. Cook until sweet potatoes are tender.

Serving Method:

Serve hot, on its own or with a side salad.

BEEF AND MUSHROOM SKILLET WITH MASHED CAULIFLOWER.

Prep Time: 15 minutes

Cooking Time: 25 minutes

Ingredients:

- 1 pound ground beef
- 1 onion, chopped
- 8 ounces mushrooms, sliced
- 2 garlic cloves, minced
- 1 teaspoon dried thyme
- Salt and pepper to taste
- 1 head cauliflower, chopped

Directions:

- In a skillet, cook ground beef over low heat until browned.
- Add onion, mushrooms, garlic, thyme, salt, and pepper to the skillet. Cook until mushrooms are tender.
- Meanwhile, steam cauliflower until tender.
- Mash cauliflower to desired consistency.

Serving Method:

Serve hot, with mashed cauliflower on the side.

AIP CHICKEN SOUP WITH ROOT VEGETABLES.

Prep Time: 15 minutes

Cooking Time: 30 minutes

Ingredients:

- 1 pound chicken breast, cubed
- 1 onion, chopped
- 2 carrots, chopped
- 2 celery stalks, chopped
- 2 garlic cloves, minced
- 6 cups chicken broth
- 2 cups diced root vegetables (such as turnips, parsnips, and sweet potatoes)
- 1 teaspoon dried thyme
- Salt and pepper to taste

Directions:

- In a large pot, combine chicken, onion, carrots, celery, garlic, chicken broth, root vegetables, thyme, salt, and pepper.
- Bring to a boil, then reduce heat and simmer for 20-30 minutes, or until vegetables are tender and chicken is cooked through.

Serving Method:

Serve hot and garnished with fresh herbs if preferred.

TURKEY AND CRANBERRY STUFFED ACORN SQUASH.

Prep Time: 20 minutes

Cooking Time: 1 hour

Ingredients:

- 2 acorn squash, halved and seeded
- 1 pound ground turkey
- 1 onion, chopped
- 2 celery stalks, chopped
- 1/2 cup dried cranberries
- 1/2 teaspoon cinnamon
- Salt and pepper to taste

Directions:

- Preheat oven to 400°F (200°C).
- Place acorn squash halves on a baking sheet, cut side down. Bake for 40-45 minutes, or until it's soft.

- In a skillet, cook ground turkey over medium heat until browned.
- Add onion and celery to the skillet. Cook until vegetables are tender.
- Stir in dried cranberries, cinnamon, salt, and pepper.
- Spoon turkey mixture into acorn squash halves.
- Bake for 15 more minutes.

Serving Method:

Serve hot, with a side salad.

AIP MEATBALLS WITH GRAVY AND MASHED CAULIFLOWER.

Prep Time: 20 minutes

Cooking Time: 25 minutes

Ingredients:

- 1 pound ground beef
- 1/2 onion, grated
- 1 garlic clove, minced
- 1/4 cup coconut flour
- Salt and pepper to taste
- 2 cups beef broth
- 2 tablespoons coconut aminos
- 2 tablespoons arrowroot powder
- 1 head cauliflower, chopped

Directions:

- Preheat oven to 400°F (200°C).

- In a bowl, combine ground beef, grated onion, garlic, coconut flour, salt, and pepper. Mix well.
- Mould the mixture into meatballs and set them on a baking sheet.
- Bake in the preheated oven for 20-25 minutes, or until cooked through.
- Meanwhile, in a saucepan, combine beef broth, coconut aminos, and arrowroot powder. Cook over medium heat until thickened.
- Steam cauliflower until tender. Mash cauliflower to desired consistency.

Serving Method:

Serve hot, with meatballs topped with gravy and a side of mashed cauliflower.

BALSAMIC GLAZED CHICKEN THIGHS WITH ROASTED BRUSSELS SPROUTS.

Prep Time: 15 minutes:

Cooking Time: 30 minutes

Ingredients:

- 4 chicken thighs
- 1/4 cup balsamic vinegar
- 2 tablespoons olive oil
- 1 tablespoon honey (optional, omit for AIP)
- 1 teaspoon dried thyme
- Salt and pepper to taste
- 1 pound Brussels sprouts, trimmed and halved

Directions:

- Preheat oven to 400°F (200°C).
- In a bowl, combine balsamic vinegar, olive oil, honey (if using), thyme, salt, and pepper.
- Place chicken thighs in a baking dish and brush with half of the balsamic mixture.
- Place Brussels sprouts in a separate baking dish and toss with the remaining balsamic mixture.
- Bake chicken thighs for 25-30 minutes, or until cooked through.
- Bake Brussels sprouts for 20-25 minutes, or until tender and caramelized.

Serving Method:

Serve hot, with chicken thighs drizzled with any remaining glaze and Brussels sprouts on the side.

AIP SHEPHERD'S PIE WITH MASHED SWEET POTATOES.

Prep Time: 30 minutes

Cooking Time: 45 minutes

Ingredients:

- 1 pound ground beef
- 1 onion, chopped
- 2 carrots, chopped
- 2 celery stalks, chopped
- 2 garlic cloves, minced
- 1 cup beef broth

- 1 teaspoon dried thyme
- Salt and pepper to taste
- 4 cups mashed sweet potatoes

Directions:

- Preheat oven to 400°F (200°C).
- In a skillet, cook ground beef over medium heat until browned.
- Add onion, carrots, celery, and garlic to the skillet. Cook until vegetables are tender.
- Stir in beef broth, thyme, salt, and pepper. Simmer for 10 minutes.
- Move the beef mixture into a baking dish.
- Spread mashed sweet potatoes over the beef mixture.
- -Bake in the preheated oven for 25-30 minutes, or until the sweet potatoes are lightly browned.

Serving Method:

Serve hot, scooping out portions with a spatula.

KITCHEN STAPLES AIP RECIPES.

AIP BONE BROTH.

Prep Time: 10 minutes

Cooking Time: 12-24 hours

Ingredients:

- 2-3 pounds of bones (chicken, beef, or pork)
- 1 onion, quartered
- 2 carrots, chopped
- 2 celery stalks, chopped
- 2 tablespoons apple cider vinegar
- Water

Directions:

- Place bones, vegetables, and apple cider vinegar in a large stockpot.
- Cover with water and bring to a boil.
- Reduce heat and simmer for 12-24 hours, adding more water as needed.
- Strain the broth and discard solids.
- Allow the broth to cool, then store in the refrigerator or freezer.

Serving Method:

Serve as a comforting drink or use as a base for soups and stews.

AIP COCONUT MILK

Prep Time: 10 minutes

Cooking Time: None

Ingredients:

- 2 cups unsweetened shredded coconut
- 4 cups hot water

Directions:

- Place diced coconut in a blender.
- Add hot water and blend on high for 2-3 minutes.
- Squeeze out as much liquid as you can using a cheesecloth or nut milk bag.
- Store coconut milk in a sealed container in the refrigerator.

Use in cooking and baking as a dairy-free alternative to regular milk.

AIP APPLESAUCE.

Prep Time: 10 minutes

Cooking Time: 20 minutes

Ingredients:

- 4-5 apples, peeled, cored, and diced
- 1/2 cup water
- 1/2 teaspoon cinnamon

Directions:

- Place apples, water, and cinnamon in a saucepan.
- Cover and cook over medium heat for 15-20 minutes, or until apples are soft.
- Mash apples with a fork or potato masher until desired consistency is reached.
- Allow applesauce to cool before serving or storing in the refrigerator.

Enjoy as a snack or use as a sweetener in baking recipes.

AIP AVOCADO OIL MAYO.

Prep Time: 5 minutes

Cooking Time: None

Ingredients:

- 1 egg (room temperature)
- 1 cup avocado oil
- 1 tablespoon lemon juice
- 1 teaspoon mustard powder
- Pinch of salt

Directions:

- In a blender or food processor, combine egg, lemon juice, mustard powder, and salt.
- With the blender running, slowly drizzle in avocado oil until mayo thickens.
- Store mayo in a sealed container in the refrigerator.

Note: You can use as a spread or in recipes calling for mayonnaise.

AIP TIGER NUT FLOUR.

Prep Time: 10 minutes

Cooking Time: None

Ingredients:

- 1 cup tiger nuts

Directions:

- Place tiger nuts in a high-speed blender or food processor.
- Blend on high until finely ground, resembling flour.
- Store tiger nut flour in an airtight container in a cool, dry place.

Use in baking as a grain-free flour alternative.

AIP HERB SALT.

Prep Time: 5 minutes

Cooking Time: None

Ingredients:

- 1/4 cup sea salt
- 1 tablespoon of dried herbs (like thyme, rosemary, or sage)

Directions:

- Combine sea salt and dried herbs in a bowl.

-   Mix well to combine.
-   Store herb salt in an airtight container.

Use as a seasoning for meats, vegetables, and other dishes.

AIP COCONUT YOGURT.

Prep Time: 5 minutes

Cooking Time: 24-48 hours (fermentation time)

Ingredients:

-   2 cans full-fat coconut milk
-   2-3 probiotic capsules

Directions:

-   Fill a clean glass jar with coconut milk.
-   Open probiotic capsules and sprinkle the powder over the coconut milk.
-   Stir well to combine.
-   Cover the jar with a clean cloth and secure with a rubber band.
-   Allow coconut milk to ferment at room temperature for 24-48 hours, or until thickened.
-   Store coconut yogurt in the refrigerator.

Enjoy as a dairy-free yogurt alternative, topped with fruit or nuts.

AIP GHEE.

Prep Time: 10 minutes

Cooking Time: 20 minutes

Ingredients:

- 1 pound unsalted butter (grass-fed, if possible)

Directions:

- Cut butter into cubes and place in a heavy-bottomed saucepan.
- Heat over medium-low heat until butter is melted.
- Continue to cook, stirring occasionally, until butter has separated into three layers (foam on top, clear butterfat in the middle, and milk solids on the bottom).
- Remove from heat and allow to cool for a few minutes.
- Strain through a fine-mesh sieve or cheesecloth to remove milk solids.
- Store ghee in a sealed container at room temperature.

Use in cooking and baking as a dairy-free alternative to butter.

A 7-DAY HEALTHY MEAL PLAN.

Here's a 7-day healthy meal plan following the Autoimmune Protocol (AIP) diet, including breakfast, lunch, dinner, snacks, appetizers and drinks:

Day 1:

- Breakfast: Coconut Flour Porridge with sliced strawberries.
- Lunch: Salad with mixed greens, avocado, grilled chicken, and olive dressing.
- Dinner: Baked salmon with roasted sweet potatoes and steamed broccoli.
- Snack: Apple slices with almond butter.
- Drink: Herbal tea

Day 2:

- Breakfast: Sweet potato breakfast bowl with coconut flakes and chopped nuts.
- Lunch: Turkey lettuce wraps with avocado and cucumber.
- Dinner: Beef stir-fry with bok choy, mushrooms, and coconut aminos.
- Snack: Mixed Berries
- Drink: Turmeric Ginger Smoothie

Day 3:

- Breakfast: Plantain waffles with coconut yogurt and blue berries.
- Lunch: Butternut squash soup with a side salad.
- Dinner: Grilled chicken thighs with cauliflower rice and sautéed spinach.
- Snack: Mixed berries.
- Drink: Coconut water.

Day 4:

- Breakfast: Apple cinnamon muffins with coconut butter.
- Lunch: Tuna salad lettuce wraps with carrots and celery sticks.
- Dinner: Baked cod with asparagus and mashed cauliflower
- Snack: AIP-friendly trail mix (coconut flakes, pumpkin seeds and dried fruit).
- Drink: Herbal tea.

Day 5:

- Breakfast: Turmeric Ginger Smoothie with collagen peptides.
- Lunch: Chicken salad with avocado mayo, served in lettuce cups.
- Dinner: Beef stew with carrots, onions and bone broth.
- Snack: Sliced cucumbers with olive tapenade.
- Drink: Bone broth.

Day 6:

- Breakfast: Coconut Milk Chia Pudding with sliced kiwi.
- Lunch: Zucchini noodles with meatballs and marinara sauce.
- Dinner: Pork chops with roasted Brussels sprouts and sweet potatoes.
- Snack: Plantain chips with guacamole.
- Drinks: Herbal tea.

Day 7:

- Breakfast: Sweet potato hash with bacon and sautéed spinach.
- Lunch: Chicken and vegetable soup with bone broth.
- Dinner: Baked chicken drumsticks with roasted beets and green beans.
- Snack: Mixed berries with coconut cream.
- Drink: Turmeric tea.

Feel free to adjust portion sizes and ingredients based on your preferences and dietary needs. It's also a good idea to consult with a healthcare professional before starting any new diet plan, especially if you have specific health concerns or conditions.

CONCLUSION.

Congratulations on completing "The Ultimate Autoimmune Protocol Diet Cookbook"!

 As you conclude this chapter, I'd want to offer you some words of encouragement and direction as you continue your AIP journey.

Starting the AIP diet is a daring and empowering step toward a healthier lifestyle. It is not always straightforward, but keep in mind that each small change is a step in the right path. Whether you're dealing with an autoimmune condition, looking for relief from inflammation, or simply wanting to improve your general state of well-being, know that you're taking control of your health and making decisions that will benefit you in the long run.

As you move forward, remember, that the AIP diet is a lifestyle change, not a quick fix. It's about feeding your body nutrient-dense foods, listening to your body's cues, and finding balance in your life. Integrating AIP principles into your lifestyle does not have to be overwhelming. Begin by focusing on complete, unprocessed meals, then gradually introduce new recipes and ingredients to your diet.

It's also worth noting that the AIP diet is not one-size-fits-all. Listen to your body and make improvements based on how you're feeling. If you are struggling, seek help from friends, family, or medical professionals who understand what's going on.

Most importantly, be compassionate towards yourself. The AIP diet is a journey that will include ups and downs. Celebrate your accomplishments, no matter how little, and don't be too hard on yourself if you experience setbacks. Every day presents a fresh opportunity to make decisions that benefit your health and well-being.

Thank you for choosing "The Ultimate Autoimmune Protocol Diet Cookbook" to help you on your AIP journey. I hope it has inspired you to adopt healthier habits and given you the ability to take charge of your health. Remember that you are capable of tremendous feats, and your health is worth investing in. Here's to a vibrant, healthy future!

THE END!